HERE'S HOW:
HEALTH EDUCATION BY EXTENSION

HERE'S HOW:
HEALTH EDUCATION
BY EXTENSION

by Ronald S. Seaton, M.D.
and Edith B. Seaton

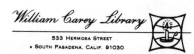

William Carey Library

533 HERMOSA STREET
• SOUTH PASADENA, CALIF. 91030

International Standard Book Number 0-87808-150-X
Library of Congress Catalog Number 76-40599

Published by the William Carey Library
533 Hermosa Street
South Pasadena, Calif. 91030
Telephone 213-799-4559

PRINTED IN THE UNITED STATES OF AMERICA

To

our children,

Douglass and Gayle

Paul and Kathy

Terry and Barbara

Jon

CONTENTS

FOREWORD

Never in history has there been a more propitious time
to unite in a single document the best thinking of the
long-separated professions of physical and spiritual
healing, and I do not doubt that Dr. Ronald Seaton and
his wife are the very best qualified team in the world
to attempt that bridge.

Ron and Edith not only possess impeccable qualifications by virtue of medical training and vast field
experience, they have also had long involvement in the
spiritual healing efforts that have been extended in
the name of Jesus Christ in the global outreach of the
Christian mission enterprise.

Over the years the physical specialists have become
increasingly aware of the essential interrelation
between their efforts and other aspects of man as an
individual and social being. As never before the same
insights are widespread among those for whom the "care
of souls" has been historically primary. Now is the

time when a book like this can foster collaboration and
understanding not only between these two helping traditions, but also between public and private initiatives.
This little book is thus welcome, timely, and most
urgently needed.

Pasadena, California   Ralph D. Winter
June 1976   Fuller Theological Seminary

PREFACE

More people in the world need health -- total health
-- than ever before. All the efforts of governments,
foundations, and missions, all their skills and their
money, their hospitals and clinics, their programs
and projects have not made the world healthier, or
solved its economic problems or its pollution problems.
The world is sicker than ever before.

Why should this be so? Perhaps it is because we
have tried to work in our own limited spheres, seeing
man as a physical body, a mind, a soul, a vote, or a
number. Every person is all of these, and more. All
of us are caught in a complex of vicious circles that
feed on themselves and strangle our uncertain attempts
to deal with crises one by one.

William and Elizabeth Paddock have written a book,
We Don't Know How, in which they seem to prove that we
really don't know how to help people help themselves
to life in all its fullness.

Is it possible to offer a functional, creative, dynamic -- healthy -- life to all? We think so. But we will need a new strategy which deals with life as a whole, and looks within each culture for the particular values and social patterns by which people live and which may need to be modified or redirected if individuals and societies are to achieve health.

Because of their concern for the whole person -- their holistic point of view -- Christian mission institutions today are uniquely qualified to initiate and sustain health promotive programs. By using members of the institution staff as trainers, mission institutions can meet the need for a cost-effective program with continuous education of those who will take the lead in bringing health to their own communities. Hospitals, schools, colleges, and seminaries can have a part in training members of each community as basic health workers to teach and to heal.

Our objective is to have each institution start at least five effective health centers a year. Some existing health projects show how this can be done. These models, as well as a pattern to be adapted to particular situations, are presented here to challenge mission agencies with a new strategy for reaching out into their communities and beyond with a life of health and wholeness.

This book was born from observation of health services in China, the United States, Korea, India, Cameroun, Kenya, Ethiopia, Egypt, Lebanon, Afghanistan, Pakistan, Nepal, Thailand, Taiwan, and Guatemala. It has grown through more than a decade of trying to give as comprehensive a health service as possible in Western India and three years of administering a wide range of health projects and institutions around the world for the United Presbyterian Church, U. S. A. It has reached maturity through an involvement in the Christian Medical Commission of the World Council of Churches and the School of World Mission at Fuller Theological Seminary.

Ideally this book should be in a looseleaf binder, because within a few years new models will update those presented here. We would not be publishing this at all if we knew that someone else had a plan for offering health, in a comprehensive sense, to a sick world. And we invite others to publish widely and share their knowledge and insights. Until someone provides a better way, out of our experience we would like to suggest: Here's How.

ACKNOWLEDGMENTS

What we know is not original with us. It is what we have learned from others modified by own own experience.

Our first acknowledgment is to those from whom we first learned, our parents, Mr. and Mrs. Luke R. Bender and Dr. and Mrs. Stuart P. Seaton. The latter, missionaries to China, are most responsible for getting us into this business in the first place.

We are indebted to the United Presbyterian Church, the United Church of Christ, and the Christian Church (Disciples of Christ) for their support while we studied and wrote.

We have been helped immeasurably by the professors at the School of World Mission of Fuller Theological Seminary: particularly Ralph Winter, who persuaded us that this book could and should be written; Charles Kraft, who guided our ventures into anthropology; and Dean Arthur Glasser, for trying to keep us on the theological straight and narrow.

We are indebted, also, to Roberta Winter for her advice and answers to our many questions about preparing the manuscript.

We acknowledge with thanks the advice of Donald Miller of Medical Assistance Programs, Inc., many of whose suggestions have been incorporated in the manuscript.

We want to acknowledge the advice and counsel, ever so gently given, of our medical friends, John Bryant, Carl Taylor, and C. S. Lewis, Jr., whose wise guidance should keep us from making some of the mistakes we have made in the past.

We express to Random House our thanks for permission to paraphrase material from *World Without Borders* by Lester R. Brown, and to the Iowa State University Press for permission to quote extensively from *We Don't Know How* by William and Elizabeth Paddock.

Finally we acknowledge the encouragement and patience of our families and friends.

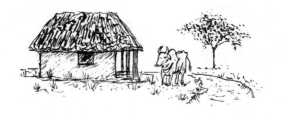

1

CAUSE FOR DESPAIR

The man who had just come into my consultation room was a friend. I passed his little shop daily as I went to and from the hospital, and we exchanged "salaams." Now he had come to the St. Luke's Hospital out-patient department complaining of fever, extreme weight loss, and coughing blood. I was shocked to see that he had far advanced and very infectious pulmonary tuberculosis.

This man's shop was on the road between the hospital and the mission school. There he sold cigarettes which he made himself, school supplies, and unwrapped peppermints which he counted out for the children from a big jar. Who could guess how many others he had infected as they stopped to chat or to buy his mints and cigarettes.

Tuberculosis is an extremely expensive illness in any society. In Third World communities the time lost from work and the cost of a prolonged hospital stay have already pauperized all but the richest families

by the time a doctor decides that surgery is a patient's
only hope.

Surgery is a last resort. The patient is usually in
poor condition. The cost to him and to the hospital is
high. It takes a great deal of the busy doctor's time
and energy, exhausts the staff, requires far more blood
than the patient's relatives and friends will give, and
depletes the hospital's meager charity funds. And if,
at such expense, one is able to "cure" a number of
serious cases of tuberculosis, he will find it is like
sewing up the hole in the grain bag after most of the
grain has spilled out. Our friend had probably
infected more people than we could take care of, even
if we could find them, and they would already be infect-
ing others. The World Health Organization estimates
that 15 million people with active tuberculosis infect
50 million more children and adolescents a year.

Many people in developing countries easily fall prey
to tuberculosis because parasites sap the vitality of
the already malnourished, keeping them from getting the
benefit of their limited food supplies. Parasite
infestation is curable, yes. But inadequate nutrition,
contaminated water, and poor sanitation start the
vicious circle all over again.

This is typical of the world's health problems. But
how can the physician, trying to cure ever larger
numbers of those who are sick -- many returning over
and over again -- leave his patients in order to get at
some of the root causes of illness by practicing preventive medicine?

CAUGHT IN INTERLOCKING CYCLES

The cycle of medical problems is only one of the
self-perpetuating downward spirals of cause and effect
that feed upon themselves, joining each other, exhaust-
ing the world's resources.

The field of economics has its vicious circle of
inflation. Workers demand higher wages. This drives
up the cost of production so that prices rise, and the
public, including the workers, suffers. Again the

workers strike for higher pay to cope with the
increased cost of living. Those who suffer most are
the people on fixed incomes, usually the poor and the
old, who have no way of adjusting to the inflated
prices.

Experts have realized for some time that food production could not increase at the same rate as the
world's exploding population. Some had seen 1975 as
the year when the food needs of the world would exceed
the amount that could be produced. This point actually
came in 1973 because of the unexpected drought causing
famine all the way from Indonesia across southern Asia,
central Africa, and even into South America. Up to
1973 the amount of food produced could have provided an
adequate basic diet for the world's people if there had
been effective and equitable distribution. Now it is
no longer possible for the earth's limited land and
water resources to supply enough food to sustain even
the present population.

In a biosphere with boundaries there is a limit to
what the land and water can produce. Pesticides help
to assure maximum yield from seed and protection for
crops, but these same chemicals flow into and contam-
inate bodies of water until they can no longer sustain
fish that can be used for food. This leads back to the
food crisis which started the cycle, with resultant
continuing damage to an ecosystem already overloaded
with mercury, lead, arsenic, cadmium, and DDT.[1]

Our consumerism and extravagant exploitation have
led to increasingly serious shortages of fish, forests,
and fossil fuels. Even after people have obtained what
they need for a relatively comfortable standard of
living they demand an increasing supply of consumer
goods. The United States, with 6 percent of the world's
population, consumes about 35 percent of the world's
total resources. While more than one billion people
live in absolute poverty, without even the basic
necessities of life, much less any luxuries, our
businesses advertise "what to buy for the man who has
everything."

In 1850 the per capita income for industrializing
countries was twice that of the rest of the world; in

1960 it had grown to fifteen times as much. By the
year 2000 the industrialized countries are expected to
have a per capita income thirty times that of less
developed nations. Between 1960 and 1970 the average
annual per capita income rose $10 in developing
nations and $300 in the more developed countries. The
average U. S. per capita income in 1970 was $4,100 (the
world's highest), while over one-half the world's
population lives on a per capita income of less than
$100 a year (Brown 1972:42-43). Yet the United States
ranks fourteenth of the sixteen most developed nations
in percentage of gross national product given as
economic assistance to the less developed nations
(McNamara Sept. 28, 1973), and the total amount of
U. S. aid to poorer countries is only moderately
larger than the New York City welfare budget (Brown
1972:49).

It is estimated that the world can sustain a gross
world product of only $6 trillion, but to raise the
entire world consumption to current United States
standards would require a gross world product of $18
trillion -- three times the world's total capacity
(Brown 1972:35, 56). Between 1950 and 1970 the gross
world product nearly tripled, reaching almost $3
trillion (Brown 1972:31). Because of such rapid
exploitation of the world's resources, economic growth
all over the world is approaching its maximum. With
the rich-poor gap between nations continually widening,
the rich can only get richer at the expense of the
poorer (Brown 1972:43). This makes it impossible for
the poor to catch up unless either they take from the
rich or the rich learn to share.

Limits to the productivity of the land led to a
rural to urban to suburban migration. By 1985 all
arable land will be under cultivation, with an additional one billion people on the earth (Freudenberger
1972). In many countries there is not sufficient land
per person for farmers to earn a living, so there is a
rapidly increasing rural to urban flow of people.

There are, of course, many things that attract
people to life in the city, not the least of which are
the better health facilities there. An added problem
related to the general rural to urban movement is

the constant migration of health personnel away from rural areas.

Because health services are inadequate in the rural parts of some developing countries where up to 80 percent of the people live, governments try hard to train doctors and nurses who will stay and work in the villages and small towns. In some countries it is a military-equivalent obligation for doctors and nurses to serve in a rural area for several years. However, almost inevitably, higher salaries, better educational facilities for children, and more social amenities tempt health personnel back into larger cities, increasing existing urban health services but leaving the rural areas without medical care.

The rural to urban flow takes place in developing countries at a rate of 5 to 8 percent per year. In 1920 about 28 percent of the world's people were city dwellers. This figure had risen to 41 percent in 1960, and will be more than 60 percent in the year 2000 (Brown 1972:84).

This great influx puts such a strain on food and water supplies, housing, sanitation facilities, and schools that a city may become practically uninhabitable. But even more people flock to the cities if these systems are improved, until they become strained again. Crowding leads to unemployment, which has now reached more than 15 percent of the labor force in India, Pakistan, Sri Lanka (Ceylon), Malaysia, and the Philippines (Brown 1972:59). Unemployment means poverty, and poverty breeds crime, prostitution, and drug abuse. Cities have become our most challenging social frontiers.

Even at the present time large, crowded cities are increasingly threatened with "unsatisfactory air quality." Air pollution leads to emphysema, bronchitis, and lung cancer. Tokyo police breathe oxygen every two hours to prevent carbon monoxide poisoning. Los Angeles children are warned against vigorous outdoor play in heavy smog (Brown 1972:18). Rotterdam has an emergency evacuation plan for the time when the city's air quality may become intolerable (Brown 1972:8).

No wonder city dwellers move back out of the cities into suburbs and beyond. But crime and drugs are accompanying them. The problems of the cities cannot be left behind. A study of some growing United Presbyterian churches in 1971 listed issues that concern many urban societies:

> . . . high suicide rate; high divorce rate; absence of the male from the home; promiscuity; boredom; the lack of any sense of community; pressures to achieve; lack of interracial contacts; excessive drinking; the drug culture; rising taxes; the generation gap; commuter frustrations; declining educational standards; the problems when both parents work; infidelity . . . . (United Presbyterian Church in the U.S.A., May, 1971).

Throughout the world 1000 persons commit suicide every day, with ten times as many attempting it. Suicide has become the second ranking cause of death for Americans between the ages of fifteen and twenty-four. The first ranking is accidents, many of which psychologists claim are due to a death wish. In Finland one of every three deaths among college students is a suicide.

Senator Walter Mondale (D., Minn.) estimates that every year one million young Americans run away from home, 6 percent of high school youth have experimented with heroin-like hard drugs, and one of every nine young people will have been in juvenile court by the age of eighteen. The most appalling estimate, by New York's Lenox Hill Hospital, is that 50,000 American children die annually as victims of child abuse, and 300,000 more are permanently injured by their parents (Lennox Hill Hospital, August, 1973). Dr. J. Corbet McDonald, at a meeting of the International Planned Parenthood Association revealed that throughout the world, because of unwanted conceptions, "nearly one pregnancy in three is deliberately terminated."

POVERTY BY OVERPOPULATION

Most of the problems societies have to face are directly related to the population explosion. In our overpopulated world the majority of the people are chronically hungry and malnourished. Nutritional deficiencies predispose people to diseases they should be able to resist. Children may become easy victims of diarrhea, measles, and pneumonia from which they would otherwise rapidly recover (Brown 1972:89). In some countries one-half the children will not live until their sixth birthdays. When expectant mothers or infants do not receive adequate protein, the chil--dren lead impaired lives from permanent brain damage and stunted bodies (Brown 1972:90).

Each case of dysentery costs a developing nation an average of twenty manpower days; malaria, thirty-five days. Tuberculosis, to which resistance is so greatly lowered by malnutrition, is the most costly of all prevalent diseases in terms of lost productivity. This loss of manpower and energy results in under production of food and more malnutrition, to the detriment not only of the nation concerned, but of the whole world whose population will nearly double in the next generation.

The so-called "Green Revolution" was the basis of a great deal of early optimism. Many hoped that the miracle grains would be able to meet the demands of a doubling population until more sophisticated technology could catch up again. But the Green Revolution has been a failure. An editorial in the Pasadena, California, *Star News* (September 27, 1973) suggests the reason:

Like most revolutions undertaken without full understanding of what would be accomplished, the Green Revolution, which was supposed to have solved the problem of world hunger, has been a dismal flop.

At the beginning of the '70s it was proclaimed that new varieties of rice, wheat, and corn would yield thrice as much food per acre as the old strains. Thus underdeveloped nations,

provided with tons of seed by the United States,
would be able to feed themselves.

What went wrong? Marvin Harris, a Columbia
University anthropologist, has given part of the
answer in two devastating reports in the magazine
Natural History (June 1972 and March 1973):

"If the new seeds are merely substituted for
local varieties," he reported, "an immediate and
drastic decline in output per acre ensues. The
so-called miracle seeds are only more productive
if they are planted in conjunction with optimum
levels of irrigation water, chemical fertilizers,
and pesticides."

This evaluation confronts us with stark realities.
Other examples could be given of early optimism giving
way to pessimism, but these may suffice to show how
mankind is trapped in many self-perpetuating interrelated cycles which have already caused the quality of
life throughout the world to deteriorate.

We cannot overemphasize the fact that the population
explosion contributes most to these worldwide problems.
It took 2 million years for the population on this
planet to reach one billion, but only 100 years more
for it to increase to 2 billion. The population of the
world is now nearly 4 billion and will be over 6
billion in 1995 (Brown 1972:134).

There are many cogent reasons for this explosion
above and beyond that of "death control" by modern
health care. A corollary to the malnourishment-
underproduction-malnourishment cycle is the amazing
fact that undernourished societies have a higher reproduction rate and consequently less food available per
capita.

One reason for the higher reproductive rate is the
need of parents in most cultures to have someone to
support them in their old age. Without pensions and
social security, they need sons to live with. Computer
statistics show that a mother in India must conceive
6.3 children to assure a 95 percent chance of having
one son alive when his father reaches sixty-five.

In developing societies, it has been said, "nutrition is an excellent contraceptive" (Brown 1972:141). So are preventive medicine, public health, and an economic growth rate of 7 to 11 percent per year. When South Korea, Japan, Taiwan, Hong Kong, and Singapore reached the goals of adequate food and economic growth a few years ago, their birth rates started to drop sharply (Brown 1972:152). Recent studies suggest that programs of social justice in particular localities may lead to a decline in birth rates, while birth rates remain high where growth is not governed by social justice.

Another means of motivating societies to moderate their population is through literacy. This is very important for family planning, but literacy and family planning programs have been losing ground in many parts of the world. There are over 700 million illiterate adults in the world -- more than ever before -- and the numbers are ever increasing (Brown 1972:114). The U. S. A. spent $839 per person on education in 1970, but India could afford only $5 per person in the same year (Brown 1972:127).

Undernourished, illiterate societies with the most inadequate health services suffer most from the population explosion. This is the half of the world living on only 7 percent of the gross world product in what Robert McNamara called absolute poverty, "a condition of life so degrading as to insult human dignity" (McNamara Sept. 28, 1973). These are the people who, as long as more privileged societies maintain their present level of demand for consumer goods, will never have the chance to achieve human dignity.

McNamara argued strongly for development assistance, citing the need for:

. . . expansion of trade, the strengthening of international stability, and the reduction of social tensions.

But . . . the fundamental case for development is a moral one.

The whole of human history has recognized the
principle -- at least in the abstract -- that the
rich and the powerful have a moral obligation to
assist the poor and the weak (McNamara Sept. 28,
1973).

Most of those able to read this book are among or in
some way related to the rich and powerful. Almost
everyone willing to read it must care, to some extent,
about those 2 billion persons who have little hope of
human dignity.

In their very convincing book, *We Don't Know How*,
William and Elizabeth Paddock state:

Malthus' "Dismal Theorem" said essentially that
if the only check on the growth of population is
starvation and misery, then no matter how favorable the environment or how advanced the technology, the population will grow until it is
miserable and starves. Kenneth Boulding has,
however, what he calls the "Utterly Dismal
Theorem." This is the proposition "that if the
only check on growth of population is starvation
and misery, then any technological improvements
will have the ultimate effect of increasing the
sum of human misery as it permits a larger proportion to live in precisely the same state of
misery and starvation as before the change."
When such a thing as a Green Revolution occurs,
its name will be Disaster if it arrives ahead
of a Population Control Revolution (Paddock and
Paddock 1973:249, 250, by permission).

BEGINNING TO LEARN

This is part of the dilemma we face in today's
world, but we do not entirely agree with the Paddocks
who conclude in the same book:

First, development professionals do not know
how to carry out an effective economic development program, either a big one or a small one.
No one knows how -- not the U. S. Government,
not the Rockefeller Foundation, not the

international banks and agencies, not the
missionaries. I don't know how. You don't
know how. No one knows how.

Second, we don't know that we don't know how
. . .

We have no knowledge of our own ignorance
(Paddock and Paddock 1973:300).

We do not entirely agree because, for one thing, the
Paddocks have now taught us a great deal about our own
ignorance. Furthermore, many of us have known for some
time that we didn't know how, but we are beginning to
learn.

We can see that the problems of the world will not
be solved as easily as we would like and had hoped.
The problems are interrelated and growing in complexity
because they repeatedly feed on themselves in vicious
circles. These circles cannot be broken by solutions
applied only one at a time in hit-or-miss fashion. A
society readily makes adaptations to short-circuit
attempts to block the momentum of existing cultural
patterns. Uncoordinated efforts are eventually phased
out for lack of permanent support.

Many programs attempting to promote health and
improved living or working conditions have been operating with no interrelationship and are often even
counterproductive to each other. Examples are numerous:

Malaria, smallpox, and measles eradication programs
where there are no family planning programs can simply
increase the number of malnourished, miserable people.

Agricultural development programs without population
planning merely add to the number of people who must be
fed.

Family planning where there are no maternal-child
health care facilities will never be accepted by a
society in which children are old-age insurance.

Nutrition education without sanitation and other preventive health measures leads only to better nourished intestinal parasites.

Hospitals and clinics that do not give health education and patient follow-up can provide only temporary cures and will find their patients returning again and again.

Health profile surveys or case finding without follow-up public health projects may frustrate all future development efforts.

Agriculture, village industry, and other self-help schemes to form cooperatives, credit unions, and marketing organizations without instruction and motivation in personal integrity can destroy the credibility of all future attempts at education for self-development.

Health education without access to health promotive programs is useless.

Public health projects without curative medical backup services are quickly discredited.

Health care facilities planned and built in rural areas without personnel available who have the moral motivation or discipline to continue serving there after government obligations have been fulfilled waste money and leave the public disillusioned and bitter.

IS HEALTH POSSIBLE?

It is only as all of these health and life promotive programs develop together in proper balance that we can accomplish what we have been told we don't know how to do.

Making health attainable for a majority of the world's people who are hungry and malnourished and receive no adequate health care appears impossible (Brown 1972:321). Some would either give up or take the rationalized but restricted advice of the Paddocks

To make hillside farming in Honduras profitable
let us first learn how to solve the problem of
subsistence farming in Appalachia . . . .

To provide housing in restless Bombay, let us
first learn how to rebuild our own ghettos.

To serve the medical needs of Ecuadorian Indians,
let us first learn to provide medical care to
the Indians in Arizona.

To eradicate malaria in Ceylon, let us first
learn how to eliminate gonorrhea in Los Angeles
. . . .

To make the wheat farmers of India competitive
with the world, let our cotton growers first
learn how to farm without subsidies . . . .

To help control the inflation which hobbles
development in Indonesia, let us first learn
how to control it at home . . . .

To make literacy a development resource in
Costa Rica, let us first learn how to profitably
employ the unskilled among our own population.

To eliminate hunger in the world let us first
learn how to improve the diets of the 5 million
Americans who cannot afford the food they need
(Paddock and Paddock 1973:303).

In a way the Paddocks are right. When the world's
problems are so complex and interrelated, it may be
wisest to commence working on them in our own back yard.
But why this preoccupation with just our own problems?
If we wait until we solve all of ours, we will never
get around to working with others on theirs. In fact,
if we fail to help others, their problems will over-
whelm us before we can solve ours. Before we finish
landscaping our property, the neighborhood will have
become a slum. As McNamara has said:

It is true that some citizens of developed
countries protest against increasing their

assistance to developing countries because of
poverty in their own societies.

They do so because they fail to distinguish
between relative and absolute poverty, or perhaps because they are obscuring the truth even
from themselves -- unwilling to admit that the
principal pressures on the incremental incomes
of their economies comes not from a legitimate
concern for societies but from the endless
spiral of their own demands for additional consumer goods (MaNamara Sept. 28, 1973).

Lester Pearson, former Prime Minister of Canada,
said, "There is a need for a revolution in mankind's
thinking as basic as the one introduced by Copernicus
who first pointed out that the earth was not the center
of the Universe" (Brown 1972:338, 339). Our thinking
about health will have to undergo a radical transformation if health is to be available to everyone. We
do know how. Whether we care enough to give up the
self-centeredness that demands more and more of the
world's goods and begin to work for the good of the
world remains to be seen.

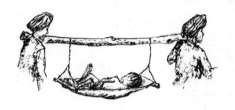

2

WHAT IS HEALTH?

Several men arrived at the hospital from a village carrying a patient in a cradle-like litter suspended from a pole. The patient was a young boy, his abdomen tender and distended from parasitic intestinal obstruction, perforation, and peritonitis. A girl in the same condition might not have been brought to the hospital at all. Her place in the economy is not so vital.

The boy had several round burns in the skin of the upper abdomen where the local village counter-irritant treatment had been tried. There were old scars there, too, signifying previous treatments for chronic abdominal pain that had resolved spontaneously. More than 95 percent of the people in this area have one sort or another of potentially dangerous intestinal parasites -- ascaris, amoebae, ancylostomes.

After trying other village remedies of herbs or oils, and probably several penicillin injections from a local medical practitioner, the family had gone to consult a priest, who may or may not have approved of our hospital. Only after all other remedies had been tried and had failed, and the boy was in desperate condition, had they brought the child to us.

We could see ashes and bits of rice the priest had applied to the boy's forehead -- the part of the body that determines one's future. The child's face was smudged with charcoal to protect him from the "evil eye." He had a charm tied to a string around his neck. A Hindu *mantra* (sacred verse) in a small silver capsule was tied to his upper arm for protection from evil spirits. A piece of string around the abdomen -- a string which would have to be removed before an operation -- remained from the child's naming ceremony when he was ten days old. A peacock feather (for good luck) tied to an ankle would have to be taken off in order to get an adequate intravenous "cut-down" started.

Families in modern India readily give consent for the removal of whichever of such amulets it is necessary to cut away, but this is because their coming to the hospital at all is a last resort indicating that they have finally reached the point of entrusting all responsibility for their critically ill relative to our doctors and nurses.

What are the basic problems that caused this child's illness and his coming to us so late? Poor sanitation; unprotected water supply; protein-carbohydrate malnutrition; lack of vitamins; and delay resulting from general ignorance, irrelevant indigenous treatment, ambiguous advice by priests, inadequate medical care, false expectations with each procedure, transportation difficulties, and an underlying fatalism -- these are just a few of the obstructions on the road to health.

Much of the world is so sick some think it is beyond help, that it is inevitable for certain parts to wither and die because of insufficient resources to sustain life. Others feel that perhaps if the sickest parts go untreated and die quickly, the rest will have a better chance to survive; a few have even suggested wiping out certain areas in order to give others a new start. But there are some who believe that the world's sickness is not hopeless and that our goal is not survival for some but health for all.

THE FOURTH DIMENSION

The World Health Organization defines health as more than the absence of disease; it is "a state of complete physical, mental, and social well-being." This is true as far as it goes, but while health is not only the absence of disease -- not only freedom from the limitations of congenital abnormalities, malignant tumors, noxious agents, microbial invasion, injury, malnutrition, faulty habits, unproductive tensions, and inadequate personal relationships -- it is also not a static state of equilibrium which might give a euphoric sense of well-being. And the WHO definition omits a fundamental dimension of human life.

Since the dawn of the human race people have been searching for some eternal meaning and purpose in life. This is the spiritual dimension which is as basic as the physical, mental, and social. Walter Goldschmidt, a past president of the American Anthropological Association, points out that in spite of the great cultural diversity of mankind, "people are more alike than cultures," and among universal human problems there is the search for some kind of symbolic eternity sought by "religious belief, good works, descendants" (Goldschmidt, 1966).

Our definition of health must include the spiritual aspect of life. This is recognized by the American Medical Association in its Department of Medicine and Religion. It is clearly indicated in the official report of the meeting of Ministers of Health of the Americas in October 1972:

It is today accepted that health is an end for each human being and a means for the society to which he belongs.

It is an end, an object of continuing individual concern, because it enables each person to realize his potential. It has been rightly said that we are what our genetic inheritance makes us and our environment allows us to be. In this context, health is a manifestation of the inate and acquired adaptive capacity of each person . . . .

It is a means, because it constitutes a component
of development, i.e., of a combination of efforts
to achieve social well-being. This is far more
than the sum of such factors as economic growth,
institutional reforms, and structural change,
among others. While all these are very important,
they fail to take account of what is for us the
essential element: the spiritual significance of
health, regarded by some as the *sine qua non* of
individual happiness.

Our definition must also see man as a whole. In the
discipline of human ecology we study total man in his
total environment, implying that human life cannot be
divided into the traditional categories of body, mind,
and spirit. Man is now scientifically conceived of
and studied as a whole. When he is whole, he is
healthy, and according to Carl Diehl, "to become whole,
man must be integrated into a community and ultimately
[into] mankind and creation" (Diehl April, 1965). At
the very minimum this brings to scientific medicine the
insistence that

> . . . sickness and healing function in at least
> four interlocking spheres: physical, mental,
> social, and spiritual; that any given illness
> may have many causes -- somatic, psychic, con-
> stitutional, genetic, social, cultural, relig-
> ious. Man's beliefs about himself and his
> environment determine to a large extent the
> interpretation of the concept of health and
> disease that governs his response to life
> crises and determine the method of therapy to
> be used in resolving them (Almquist April,
> 1967:5).

We can say, then, that *health is a dynamic state of
physical, mental, social, and spiritual integration
enabling achievement of the maximum potential in all
of human life.* This is a functional definition which
gives us a sense of direction (dynamic integration of
all human dimensions) and a creative approach to the
optimal quality of human life (realizing the maximum
potential of any person or group of persons).

Having arrived at a definition of health, we now explore the conditions which must be fulfilled to achieve it.

UNIVERSAL IMPERATIVES

Physiologists, psychologists, and anthropologists list fifteen basic needs -- "universal imperatives" -- which are found in all cultures and without which communities of human beings do not long survive.(2) These are:

Primary needs
1. Clean air, food, and water
2. Elimination of wastes
3. Sleep
4. Protection from climate
5. Security
6. Sex and reproduction
7. Freedom from disease

Derived needs
1. A sense of belonging to family or other social group
2. Communication
3. Social organization

Integrative needs
1. Dignity (a sense of personal worth)
2. Meaning and purpose in life
3. A sense of values or guidelines for living
4. Aesthetic expression
5. Recreation

Although these are basic and universal requisites for healthy individuals in a healthy society, the way in which they are supplied and integrated will vary from culture to culture. The value placed on various needs and the part each plays is determined by a particular society's own beliefs and knowledge -- what Keesing and Keesing call the "world view" (Keesing and Keesing 1971:Chap. XV), and Ruth Benedict in *Patterns of Culture* identifies as "cultural configuration" (Benedict 1934:Chap. VII).(3) For example, even to

enumerate basic needs suggests a world view with a
Western orientation. Mahlon M. Hess has noted that

> . . . while Westerners tend to compartmentalize
> their lives, to the Oriental and to primitives
> life is a unified whole. Providing the material
> necessities of life, social relations with one's
> own group and with those outside the group, per-
> petuation of the family and the culture, and
> relations with the supernatural are regarded as
> being, as indeed they are, intertwined and inter-
> dependent (Hess 1957:170-184).

Our Western secularized culture differs from most of
the others in this respect. Our Greek heritage has
left us with a pragmatic and pluralistic concept of the
universe. Aristotle once argued about "whether moral
law or medicine is nobler; whether it is a higher goal
to make men virtuous or to make them sound of health"
(Fletcher 1954:4). This has led Western civilizations
to their present high degree of specialization and
scientific achievement. It even led us for a long
time to consider the individual as being divided into
body, mind, and soul. But recent progress in psycho-
somatic medicine compels us to modify a "world view"
that regards the human body as merely a set of separate
parts.

What is true of the individual in this sense is true
of creation as a whole. Computers have been able to
integrate the huge masses of information that specialists have collected in order to achieve spectacular
scientific feats in space and nuclear physics. This
should not surprise us, as scientists and philosophers
now agree on the basic unity of all that exists in this
universe.

> As twentieth century scholarship advanced, the
> longstanding tendency to treat elements of
> experience as if they had an objective unit
> existence began to show major inadequacies.
> Our Western languages gave difficulty here,
> for they were filled with unit concepts and
> contrasts: mind and matter, body and soul,
> time and space, atoms, chemical elements,
> behavioral traits. Such a new and necessary

point of view as Einstein's relativity theory not only shook the scientific world but also bulged beyond familiar language symbols.

The newer frame of reference, carried partly on fresh concepts, emphasized the interrelations of elements of experience, and the significant combinations of elements comprising whole systems. By the 1920s and 1930s every field of knowledge from science to philosophy was being strongly affected by these viewpoints. In the philosophy of science, for example, A. N. Whitehead (as in his *Science and the Modern World*, 1926) called it "holistic," "integrative," "functional" in the sense that all the parts of a system *do* something, that is, have a significant function in relation to the whole. In psychology, as many will know, the so-called Gestalt psychology broke in vigorously upon the older types of behaviorism (Keesing and Keesing 1971:387, 388).

It is this organismic, holistic (wholistic), integrative, functional concept that we want to stress in our approach to promoting health. In formulating principles to achieve individual and community health we will deal here with integrating in a holistic, functional way the basic and imperative human needs. Benjamin Paul and Walter Miller say in *Health, Culture and Community*:

It would simplify matters if personal and community health could be isolated and treated apart from the complexities of local existence . . . . Health practices and health ideas penetrate deeply into the domains of politics, philosophy, etiquette, religion, cosmology, and kinship . . . . Health workers would do well to adopt a way of looking at the community that gives some coherence and depth to the array of observable details. No one frame of reference can fully serve this purpose, but the concept of culture fills part of the need (Paul 1955:460).

In an organismic sense, it is not possible for one
part of a community or culture to be unhealthy and the
other parts to be securely healthy any more than for
one organ or limb to be diseased and the rest of the
body unaffected. This fact has been demonstrated
repeatedly in history. It is being demonstrated
universally now in the arenas of urban confrontation
and world politics. It is the supreme argument against
any kind of isolationism, whether in a family, a community, or a country. People can be psychologically or
socially healthy only within a healthy cultural framework. As John Donne said, "No man is an island, entire
of itself . . . . any man's death diminishes me" (Donne
1970:453). Secretary of State Henry Kissinger summed
it up by saying that the common interest is also everyone's self-interest. We are our brother's keepers --
for our own health.

Since we have defined health as a dynamic state of
physical, mental, social, and spiritual integration
enabling achievement of the maximum potential in all of
human life, it is obvious that a culture's world view
as it attempts to explain, validate, reinforce, and
integrate the total range of beliefs and behavior in
cultural patterning is vitally important to health.

Problems occur when innovations which are imperative
for the health of individuals or communities don't
immediately fit into the world view, because this
arouses questions about the validity of that particular
cultural configuration. For example, a group of Kilba
in Northern Nigeria practice infanticide, permitting
death by exposure of babies born to unmarried girls who
are required to prove their fertility before marriage
(Kraft 1973:172), and in certain parts of India
infanticide has been practiced when a child is born
after its father has died.

On one occasion a man bitten by a snake was taken to
be treated by the priest in a Hindu temple. When the
man died the priest sent a message to the mission
hospital doctor: Please come and start this man's
heart so that I can cure him. A doctor in the same
hospital had succeeded in saving a woman bitten by a
cobra. When the woman was obviously recovering her
relatives came to the doctor to ask whether they might

now release the snake. They had kept the cobra alive
in a clay pot, since they believed killing the snake
would cause the woman's death. Now they planned to
release it in the same field where it had bitten the
woman. Eventually world views with such customs will
have to adapt or change in order to integrate the
necessary healthy innovations.

In working with people toward improving their health
it is essential to start where they are. The innovations must be relevant to the culture and easily
appropriated. We must search for the cultural forms
and use these to communicate in health education and
application. For example, in many developing countries
the phases of the moon are important for social and
religious reasons. It will be possible to time women's
28-day cyclic contraceptives to match both their
rhythms and the moon's. We must, however, remain free
enough of cultural pressures to be sure that certain
families or communities do not lead a program into
restricted diversions of vested interest that obviously
are not beneficial to all, or more particularly, to the
most deprived.

HOW DO WE MEASURE HEALTH?

What are the criteria by which we measure the health
of an individual or a society?

Physically there must be utilization of optimal
levels of productive energy. This depends on adequate
nutrition, homes, sanitation, protected water supplies,
medical and dental facilities for preventive and curative care, and maternal-child health and family planning
services. Along with these individuals must have a
freeing sense of security, self-knowledge, accurate
perception, honest expression, and adequate response
(Lapsley 1972:112). The health of individuals and
communities is evaluated by their sense of social
equity and justice controlled by mercy, discipline,
freedom, and integrity within a framework of mutual
concern. There is perhaps no better indicator of health
in a holistic sense than the extent to which the lives
of persons demonstrate the characteristics enumerated
in Paul's letter to the Galatians 5:22-23: love, joy,

peace, patience, kindness, goodness, faithfulness,
gentleness, and self-control.

If the world view of any culture does not permit
reaching the maximum potential in human life in all of
these areas, it needs to be transformed so that each
individual and social unit in it may be as healthy as
possible. A study of anthropology suggests how this
can be done.

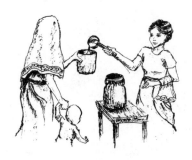

3

HEALTH EDUCATION BY EXTENSION

At St. Luke's Hospital we had a very large well-baby clinic. Well-baby clinic was what it was meant to be, but many of the children who came were sick.

There were two main inducements for mothers to bring their children to the clinic -- free medical examinations and distribution of powdered milk. But we learned that when we ran out of milk, the clinic attendance dropped precipitously, and we often wondered what was happening to the many sick children who were brought in only when we had milk to give out.

We learned that the same child would be sick again and again, frequently with the same disease. It did not matter how much we explained to the mother about preventive health care. Nor did it matter how well the child was on leaving the hospital after he had been admitted for an acute critical illness.

We learned that no matter how hard we tried to control the distribution, the milk often went into the family's tea, rather than only to the children.

We learned that when a child was sick, the problems
were usually multiple. There was the mother's
inability to make the preventive health adjustments in
her home or to change unhealthy habits or customs; the
failure to have the children seen at the clinic when
there was no milk powder, and the lack of integrity in
the use of milk given to the children; the continued
grinding poverty; the unwillingness to plan for fewer
children, or even for the spacing of the children; and
the community's inability to supply clean water or
adequate sanitation. Almost invariably malnutrition
and intestinal parasites were part of the disease
complex. Hunger is the most widespread of all the
world's health problems. Ascariasis is practically
universal in developing countries.

IS WORLD HEALTH POSSIBLE?

In 1973 the World Health Organization estimated the
number of cases of the most prevalent diseases in the
world as follows (Martin, April 7, 1973): hookworm,
450 million; trachoma, 400 million; filariasis, 200
million; schistosomiasis, 200 million; onchocerciasis,
30 million; tuberculosis, 15 million; leprosy, 11
million; Chagas disease, 7 million. These diseases
appear mostly in underdeveloped countries. Cardio-
vascular diseases, cancer, environmental pollution,
accidents, mental illnesses, deficiency diseases, and
drug abuse are also widespread. The task of providing
health to the world is immense.

WHO has found, however, that to provide adequate
health services in both the developed and developing
countries there are insufficient funds, poor structur-
ing of the health services, shortage of trained staff,
poor utilization of available staff and funds, and
concentration on short term rather than long term
needs (WHO Executive Board Report, 1973). It is for
this state of affairs that, from a holistic point of
view, we will suggest corrective principles.

MOTIVATION -- FROM OUTSIDE AND INSIDE

With many of the basic human needs constantly "felt" by at least two-thirds of the world's people, we would hardly be surprised if some had to be restricted from meeting their own needs by force at the expense of their neighbors. Am I not justified in taking some of your grain if my family is starving, or seizing your barn if I have no house?

Yet even among the world's suffering two-thirds, some of whom have never known a day without hunger or sickness, many are not sufficiently aware of exactly what their needs are or of the potential for helping themselves with what resources are immediately available to them. Some even seem to be numbed into inaction and hopelessness by constant nagging needs. Many live in peasant villages which, as George M. Foster points out, are part of economically depressed nations, so that other parts of the country cannot provide much help. Technical services are often poor or lacking altogether. As Foster says, it is not "that community development is unsuccessful; it is good, and sometimes excellent . . . . The point is that a *conceptual* and *philosophical* cultural fit are essential in defining programs . . . ." (Foster 1973:183).

The world view or total perspective of people in a particular culture is studied by examining their beliefs, folklore, customs, and behavior patterns. From these we learn how people are motivated to change. Motivation begins with what Paulo Freire calls *concientización* -- self awareness or self-knowledge -- and leads through interests, evaluation, and trial to adoption and confirmation or non-adoption and discontinuance. But the beginning is an awareness of basic information.

There are in all cultures many different motivating forces which we can learn and legitimately use without being subtly manipulative. In addition to certain of the imperative basic needs already mentioned there are other motivating forces. These may develop spontaneously in a society receptive to innovation, or they may be offered as incentives to promote changes. Among them are:

1. Anticipation of a practical *reward* to a *felt* need. (The reward may be only a promise to "solve a problem," but the more immediate the reward the better.)
2. Desire for special recognition or prestige.
3. Relief from oppression, fears, or prejudice.
4. Stimulation by suitable innovators.
5. Interest through education.
6. Capability of understanding new ideas.
7. Freedom to enquire and act.
8. Anticipation of change.
9. Support from favorable opinion.
10. Competition and pride in family, community or nation.
11. Obligation of friendship.
12. Suitability. Any change or innovation must "fit" into the "way of life," the "philosophy," the "basic beliefs and values," the "world view" that all people tend so universally to defend.(4)

It is clear that motivation will have to come from the perspective of those living in a particular culture.

In Barnett's terminology, though an outsider may "advocate" a change, only the members of a society may "innovate" for that society. That is, how the cultural patterning is to be used -- whether for the perpetuation, alteration or replacement of the present practice -- is up to the members of the culture or group in question alone. An outsider, though he may appeal for change, is limited to his ability to win over some insider who will then effect the change(s) from within (Kraft 1973:172).

According to Kraft "the advocate who aims at effective transformational change should seek to encourage a minimum number of critical changes in the world view rather than a larger number of more peripheral changes (Kraft 1973:426). He must seek to cure the disease rather than merely to treat the symptoms. A "conceptual transformation" can never be imposed from outside upon either an individual or a culture.

Kraft insists that the external advocate of change
must seek to understand, without necessarily agreeing
with, the point of view of people whose cultural
patterning may need change. Paul and Miller agree:

If you wish to help a community improve its
health, you must learn to think like the people
of that community . . . . What appears from the
outside as irrational belief and behavior
becomes intelligible when viewed from within
(Paul and Miller 1955:1, 4).

The means by which an advocate is able to perceive
and to influence for good is love, which Eugene Nida
defines as "a profound appreciation of the worth and
value of people as God sees them." This love is "the
only transforming power in the world. Force may bring
conformity, but only love can transform the heart
. . . . A man who is forced or bribed will in the end
inevitably turn against whatever power has so subtly
insulted his integrity. The way of love is not fast,
but it is sure . . . ." (Nida 1960:217, 218).

The advocates and innovators who seek change and
improvement should be involved in a program of continuous health extension education using all relevant
indigenous forms of communication. Whether or not this
is a cross cultural program, in order to be effective,
all agents of change must understand how and why the
people they are dealing with feel, think, and behave
the way they do. Benjamin Paul says:

To enhance the likelihood of success the educator
must modify the form of his health message so
that it makes sense to the particular audience
for which it is intended. To do this well, he
must be able to look at the world from the
other person's frame of reference. The process
of re-education is thus two-sided, applying to
the dispenser as well as the recipient of information. To teach, the health educator must be
able to learn . . . . (Paul and Miller 1955:4).

The hopeful and helpful fact is that, as Nida points
out:

(1) the processes of human reasoning are essentially the same, irrespective of cultural
diversity, (2) all peoples have a common range
of human experience, and (3) all peoples
possess the capacity for at least some adjust-
ment to the symbolic "grids" of others (Nida
1960:90).

This means that advocates and innovators can communicat
and understand each other on the basis of their common
humanity. Advocate and innovator must share, in a
spirit of complete openness, this process of introducin
new information and new values that can produce changes
in the thinking and behavior of the community. The
aim will be a "conceptual transformation" with continua
progress toward health. It may be difficult at first,
but it is possible.

It may seem that all people should be highly motivated to work toward innovations affecting their own
and their society's health. However, those whose world
view is cyclic or fatalistic may lack motivation to
change. Motivation may be especially poor when the
innovating individuals feel themselves under obligation
to or pressure from the advocates. Any form of public
service which depends on coercion or fails to develop
incentive rewards in terms of the culture's values will
result in inadequate return for the amount of input.
On the other hand, rewards appropriate to the effort
expended and related to basic or cultural felt needs
can, with proper management, give a result much greater
than the sum of all input.

The best and perhaps the only way we can get people
to make a commitment or change their habits is through
a continuous personal relationship. This is why Carl
Taylor has said that mobile health units, whether on
curative or preventive medicine missions, are not only
ineffective but can cause more harm than good unless
there is a local resident health worker to follow up
patients and continually reinforce health education.
It is the innovator within a community who can most
effectively help his people to change.

HOW DO WE START?

We have already noted that many of the world's health problems are interrelated and in self-perpetuating cycles and can be attacked effectively only on many fronts and in an integrated way.

One of our goals in developing healthy improvements is to get the maximum basic medical services on a continuous basis to the maximum number of people. These services include adequate nutrition, clean water, clean environment, dental prophylaxis, immunizations, and family planning and maternal-child health care with a basic level of treatment for the 80 to 85 percent of illnesses that are amenable to simple or repetitive measures (Sai, April, 1973).

Another goal is to achieve extended health service within the resources of structure, personnel, and funds that developing countries can afford in order to keep their infrastructures free from continuing foreign subsidies. One means of doing this is to search out, train, and encourage to remain in service all who are already delivering any kind of health care, no matter how simple it may be.

Every community has at least one person who is looked to for advice, if not actual care, in times of sickness. This may be a midwife, granny, village health worker, shaman, medicine man, witch doctor (avoiding the witch and sorcerer), priest, herbalist, health vistor, druggist, nurse's aide, practical nurse, registered practitioner, or even a local teacher or pastor. It is helpful, if possible, to avoid polarization and competition and to build on what is already available.

Ideally we would train basic health workers, teaching them to teach others how to achieve health in its broadest sense, assisting them to serve in some capacity those who are sick, and helping them to prevent illness and to promote the maximum in productivity and creativity by individuals in their own communities. The basic health workers would have a more diversified training and broader area of concern than the usual paramedic or China's "barefoot doctors" (actually

neither barefoot nor doctors) who are trained to deal
only with medical problems (Horn, 1969).

Such a health training program can best be developed
by continuous extension education. It is surprising
that extension education has not been a more prominent
part of many health services, for it makes it possible
for programs to reach the maximum number of people.
Its principles are informal person-to-person exchange
of information; studying and observing continuously
while serving in one's own community; and learning by
discovery in doing rather than by indoctrination. One
of the most effective methods of health education is
the use of programmed instruction.

Ivan Illich claims that Western education has become
inadequate for preparing people to live in these days.
He suggests "de-schooling" and non-formal education.
Others suggest that transistor radios and television
programs like "Sesame Street" can replace schools. A
satellite has been placed over India with the hope that
before long a television set can be made available in
each village for teaching and transmitting information

Radio and television can play a part in the learning
process, but adequate non-formal education requires
personal interaction, a relationship between advocate
and innovator and between innovator and community, which
transmitted monologue communication does not offer.
Even in a literate society John and Elaine Cumming four
as others have, ". . . for the health educator . . .
mass media were less effective than group contacts"
(Paul and Miller 1955:66).

Jesus is the most eminent example of teachers who
went out to where the people were. Another notable,
more recent example is John Wesley. Ralph Winter,
editor of *Theological Education by Extension*, says:

> John Wesley's method of extension training, his
> method of establishing classes and training
> . . . leaders, ought to be . . . important to
> us as an example. Meanwhile the communists have
> borrowed Wesley's training methods and cell
> structure and harnessed them to the conversion
> of the world -- to communism! How ironic that

theological education teaches his theology and
the communist movement practices his method!
The amazing flexibility and penetration of
communist cells . . . should at least open our
eyes to the importance of extension (Winter 1969:
400).

We should not let the Communists be the only ones to
capitalize on extension education.

CAN IT BE COST-EFFECTIVE?

One of the principle advantages of health training
by extension is that it can be cost-effective. Many
forms of preventive medicine or public health programs
in developing countries have been too expensive or
incapable of self-support. If a program of health
education by extension can be built upon an already
self-sustaining or otherwise permanently stable base,
it can extend out into surrounding communities without
fear of sudden collapse from a lack of support.

Too much financial backing for development projects
can be counterproductive, but a limited amount of
assistance correctly given -- whether it signals gen-
uine human concern or only raises a sense of hope --
generates an unexplainable increase in leadership and
effort with greater productivity by the recipient
community. It is not easy to strike the right balance
between too much and too little assistance. Initially
some "seed" money may be required to get a project
started, but caution should be exercised lest the program be smothered by paternalism before it can even
get off the ground. We must plan a program that over
the long haul will not require more support than a
developing country currently spends for health, in the
holistic sense, per capita per year. The amount now
being spent is probably about as much as that country
can afford. We need to be sure it will be used where
the people have no health care rather than in duplicating elite services (Bryant 1968:48).

Even in cities health services often fail to reach
the poorer masses. Within the next few decades three-
fourths of the world's population will be living in

overcrowded urban areas. Health education by extension
must reach into ghettos and slums.

If a health extension program can be cost-effective
while serving those in greatest need, it will demonstrate the possibility and desirability of repeating
it, even on a large scale. Certain types of health
insurance programs or health maintenance organizations
already in operation may be suitable for some developing countries.(5)

There are many possible kinds of support bases.
Primary health centers or district hospitals subsidized
by government funds would be appropriate. Other private or public institutions could also serve. Mission
hospitals, agriculture or technical schools, and
seminaries, all with a holistic conception of health,
could easily be adapted to conduct a program of health
education by extension. Governments, foundations,
and other organizations often give generous support to
community health programs -- especially those emphasizing family planning.

It is important that all concerned, advocating institution and innovating community, understand the advantages both derive from such programs. In a mission
hospital, for example, the administration can quickly
see how an education extension program will continually
improve public relations with surrounding communities
and increase public utilization of the medical facilities. This in turn will increase the hospital's
ability to be self-supporting and thus its opportunities to be more involved with others in community and
country development. The medical staff of a mission
hospital will find that their extended contacts
facilitate case finding of new and possibly infectious
diseases, follow-up of discharged patients to validate
or improve upon the treatment given (Thurber, 17),
opportunities for research which is directly related
to preventive medicine and public health, and possibilities for much wider involvement in family planning.

A HOLISTIC APPROACH

All extension programs in a given area, whether developed by government, mission institutions, or other voluntary agencies, must be integrated with each other in a holistic approach. John Cassel, reporting on a comprehensive health program among South African Zulus, concludes that

> . . . the improvement of health conditions cannot be conceived as an isolated effort; rather it must be seen in its total context [which] includes economic, political, and ecological considerations, as well as many features of the local culture . . . . Thorough understanding of local ways and values and the importance of fitting new ideas into the existing cultural framework of the people were shown to be essential if lasting results were to be achieved. The experiences . . . demonstrated the advantages of an integrated service wherein the promotive-preventive and curative aspects of health are combined and made the responsibility of the same team (Paul and Miller 1955:38, 40).

Valuable health services must not duplicate each other. The approach to meeting the needs indicated by preliminary surveys should be that of a team, with each participant an important member of the partnership. If a government is able to subsidize or take over certain parts of a total program, so much the better. In other areas other members of the team may start needed innovations with government permission and, if possible, assistance.

GETTING DOWN TO BASICS

It is helpful if not vital for the government to give some sort of recognition to development efforts, especially in a self-help program which stresses health education by extension. A certificate, diploma, degree, or license that confers status or rewards service rendered and problems solved or avoided may add greatly to the motivation of the innovating basic health worker.

If at all possible, the local community power structure should choose the innovator. This assures the
greatest degree of moral support if not of remuneration.
It also promises some possibility of community control.
The power structure may be political, social, economic,
religious, or military, and its cooperation helps to
guarantee that the training and innovations will pro-
ceed more efficiently.

Health education by extension requires that most of
the training be given where the basic health workers
live. This could mean that in-service, non-formal
programmed instruction might be given over single band
radios. There will be occasions when the workers
should become acquainted with and study in institutions
that offer referral services, but it is most important
that basic health workers should learn to be effective
in the situations where they serve, rather than under
unfamiliar conditions. Also they must be able to study
and learn without having to leave their families or
their regular means of earning a living. This is in
contrast to the usual resident programs of training
schools and colleges. This method permits a natural
selection for training of many kinds of people, young
and old, rich and poor, housewife and farmer, who have
a special aptitude for or interest in health work.

Because conditions -- soils, climates, diseases,
pests, customs, beliefs, languages, resources -- vary
so much even in limited areas, it is important that the
instruction materials be prepared indigenously unless
appropriate and inexpensive teaching material is
already available. Having materials prepared locally
will often decrease their cost and can give added
status to the local trainers or teachers who prepare
the necessary books or manuals.

Most important of all, the teaching must be of the
best quality possible in each situation, with advocates
trainers, teachers, supervisors, and administrators
highly motivated by a deep concern for those they seek
to serve. We must earn the right to be teachers, to
be heard. We cannot afford mistakes in matters that
involve people's livelihood and their very lives.

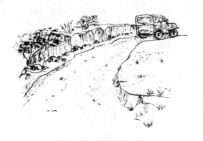

4

THE ROLE OF THE BASIC
HEALTH WORKER

We did almost everything right.

Every other week our St. Luke's Hospital team consisting of a doctor, a nurse, an evangelist, and a
driver went to the village of Tulas about eight miles
from Vengurla. The road was rough and dusty or rutted
and muddy, according to the season -- hard on the Jeep
and hard on us. We arrived hot and covered with red
dust or cold, soaked by the monsoon rains.

The village "librarian," who also had many other
official duties, had invited us to hold our clinic in
the Panchayat (elected village leaders) office which
also served as the library. We had status.

One of our friends in the village had a daughter,
an intelligent young woman who took a keen interest in
the clinic. She often watched our activities and in
the middle of the afternoon served tea to the busy
team. We had good local help.

The clinic was well attended, which surprised me
because our own hospital out-patient department was not
far away, considering the distances to some health care
facilities in India, and bus service was reasonably
good. Our volume of service was so great that the
clinic was self-supporting.

We didn't have the luxury of an X-ray machine or
lab, but we did have an adequate examining room, and we
did a fairly good job of diagnosing and of dispensing
inexpensive and reasonably effective medicines.

One day I examined a man who complained of having had
a cough and low grade fever for ten days. Through the
stethescope I heard nothing significant in his chest,
so I gave him some sulfa, soda, and cough medicine for
a mild case of pneumonia. He told me later that I had
not instructed him to come to the hospital if he didn't
improve within a few days or if he became worse. It
was our practice for the doctor or the nurse dispensing
the medicines to say this to every patient.

Two weeks later one of my colleagues was in charge
of the Tulas clinic, and my patient did not present
himself for follow-up even though, as we learned later,
he was worse. It was four weeks after I'd first seen
the patient that I went to the clinic again. At that
time some of the man's family came to ask me to see him
at his home because he wasn't able to come the quarter
mile to the clinic.

I found the man lying on a rough blanket on the
cowdung-plastered floor, dying of far advanced, dissem-
inated, and obviously highly contagious tuberculosis.
We sent the patient in the Jeep to the hospital where
he received emergency care while we finished the clinic
and followed later.

Many months later, after great expense to the hospital, to me, and to the patient's family, he returned
home well. But we had learned a costly lesson. If
only we had trained someone living in the village --
someone like the attentive young woman who was anxious
to be of service -- as a basic health worker to follow
up on our sicker patients, she could have checked their
progress, advised them what to do if there was no

improvement, and notified us before it was too late.
She could have had status as a health visitor, family
health worker, or nurse's aide, or she might even have
been trained as an auxiliary nurse-midwife. We had a
good village clinic, doing almost everything right
except teaching someone in that community how to help
us promote health.

FROM PARAMEDICS TO BASIC HEALTH WORKERS

Paramedics are not new. For many years medical
missionaries in Africa, Latin America, and Asia have
trained medical assistants, auxiliaries, dressers,
midwives, health visitors, assistant medical officers,
and various levels of nurses to work out from the
central mission institutions (Elliott, 1972). I
remember my father sending out "druggists" that he had
trained into Chinese villages where they offered a kind
of extended medical care. Communists in China learned
the concept of "barefoot doctors" from Christian missionaries.

Kenneth Scott Latourette noted that missionaries in
China "pioneered in the introduction of Western medicine, in public health education . . . ." (Latourette
1953:1326). In 1917 the Medical Missionary Association,
Y. M. C. A., and National Medical Association combined
efforts and conducted public health campaigns in a
number of areas in China (Christian Literature Society
for China 1917:418). Dr. Edward M. Dodd wrote in 1933
of the outstanding work started under mission auspices
by Dr. W. W. Peter, whom he called "the moving spirit
behind the Council on Public Health Education of China"
(Dodd 1933:7). By 1924 this council had departments for
(1) School Hygiene, (2) Child Health, (3) Community
Hygiene, and (4) Chinese Literature (Christian Literature Society for China 1924:360).

For many years medical missionaries have tried to
help developing nations cope with such major medical
problems as tuberculosis, malaria, malnutrition, intestinal parasites and infections, venereal disease,
trachoma, schistosomiasis, leprosy, filariasis, and
childhood infectious diseases. Most of their corrective measures can be found in the "S" list: sewers,

spray, screens, soap, sanitation, shoes, sufficient
food, and simple medicines.

As we have seen, however, health is more than the
absence of disease, and the basic health worker must
be more than a paramedic. In his or her concern for a
dynamic physical, mental, social, and spiritual integration of human life the scope of his activities could
include: health surveys;(7) case finding; follow-up on
leprosy(8) and tuberculosis; referrals; liason with
other development services; school health programs;
family planning;(9) first aid;(10) home deliveries;
immunizations;(11) day care centers; under-fives
clinics;(12) prenatal and postnatal care;(13) community
health education; group discussions on human values and
social justice; evangelism; instruction in nutrition;(14
health demonstration projects; water resources development;(15) maintenance of family health files;(16)
instruction in sanitation and improving waste disposal;
(17) dental prophylaxis and care; simple diagnostic
procedures;(18) symptomatic treatment;(19) routine
curative treatment (under appropriate medical supervision) for minor illnesses(20) such as simple diarrhea,
bronchitis, and malaria, with complete and accurate
records(21) to assure quality control (See Appendix A).

The disease pattern in one rural area of a rapidly
developing country shows that: 40 percent of the problems are largely due to ignorance of basic health
concepts; 70 percent can be simply diagnosed and simply
treated; 90 percent can be satisfactorily treated without a specialist; and 10 percent can be satisfactorily
treated only with care by a specialist (Thurber).
Thus most of the medical problems can come within the
range of the basic health worker's responsibility. For
example, if we can teach every midwife to flame the
knife or scissors with which she cuts the newborn's
umbilical cord, we can virtually eliminate infant
tetanus.

AN APPROACH TO MENTAL ILLNESS

Closely related to physical disease is mental
illness. Different cultures not only have different
kinds and degrees of mental illness,(22) but also

have different ways of caring for people who are mentally disturbed or disadvantaged.(23) Mental diseases can be so bizarre and mysterious that people often have deep religious interpretations of their origin and nature.

The health education teams will need to teach basic health workers to help communities accept the mentally distressed and assist them to become comfortable and contributing members of society. This may be very difficult because creating healthier attitudes will even affect the culture's world view. But it is much easier in cultures with extended families that can cope more effectively with a certain amount of abnormal behavior. Possibly most difficult for the teams to learn and teach will be how to predict and handle dangerous or self-destructive behavior.(24) Fortunately in a supportive and caring environment this problem does not occur very often.

We have said that health involves the whole of life -- that to achieve individual and community health we must integrate in a holistic, functional way the basic and imperative human needs. A single worker cannot hope to deal in depth with all the areas which affect the health of the community, but each worker must be aware of the interrelation of all dimensions of life as they pertain to total health and know where development assistance can be found.

ILLITERACY AND HEALTH

This awareness and knowledge come through an educational process. Whatever the subject matter, whether the indigenous method is formal or non-formal, education may be enhanced through the use of literary symbols, that is, written language. Yet almost one-half of the adults in the world are illiterate, and illiteracy is increasing. In Ethiopia, Afghanistan, Nepal, Saudi Arabia, Kerman, Mozambique, and Angola nearly 95 percent of the people are illiterate. Twenty other countries have an illiteracy rate of above 80 percent.

The most capable and highly motivated candidate for training as a basic health worker may be one who can't

read or write, yet governments are likely to require a
predetermined academic level before giving official
recognition to basic health worker training. The
illiterate candidate need not be disqualified. Adult
education textbooks can be prepared which include
literacy as part of the total program. When a basic
health worker passes his general education examinations
at the required level, official recognition will bring
prestige to him and to the whole program.

Literacy training included in health education may
help people to improve the quality of their lives as
they learn to use the resources available to them.
Classes in literacy may simultaneously teach about
farming, cottage industries, social values, counseling,
religion, and art.

FARMERS AND RURAL DEVELOPMENT

The lives of all of us depend on farmers, yet farmers
are perhaps the most exploited group in the world.
Health education might well begin by recognizing the
importance of the farmer and leading the community to
assure him freedom to make responsible choices. For a
farmer struggling to earn a living on a small piece of
land not his own, dignity comes with justice in land
distribution, equitable marketing opportunities, and a
part in decision making (Freudenberger, 1972). The
extension education team will realize that the small
farmer cannot take the risks involved in innovation.
One failure for him would be disastrous. The team will
first have to demonstrate new methods that will enhance
the farmer's productivity and standard of living.
Farmers need to be able to get instructions for mixing
pesticides and using proper fertilizers. They need to
know how to obtain quality seeds; where to go for
advice; how to run a credit union, set up a double-
entry bookkeeping system, market their produce.
Attention to the farmer and farming will lead to other
phases of rural development: soil testing,(25)
irrigation,(26) drainage, tools, farm power, fencing,
animal stock, fish ponds,(27) conservation and quaran-
tine laws, markets, roads, bridges, and cooperatives.

Health education by extension should provide leadership training in community organization and make community leaders acquainted with the resources and technical knowledge available through government and other organizations -- information about soil management, care of animals, collection and storage of food products.(29) It may offer guidance for building small cottage industries(29) which can move money out to rural areas so that people no longer need to flock to the cities to make a living.

For those who can read, a cheap mimeographed newsletter could provide many kinds of information. A valuable tool is the looseleaf notebook of locally prepared educational material which can be updated regularly.(30) Cassette tapes will be most helpful for not-yet-literate individuals or groups.

Health education by extension means assisting people to discover their own interests, varieties of capabilities, and local raw materials. It means teaching them to find tools, credit, and other necessary resources and outlets for their small cottage industry products. It means educators becoming partners with learners who are seeking a life of dignity and meaning. Implicit in extension training is the responsibility of each learner to help and teach others.

A HEALTHY SOCIETY

Simply raising the standard of living does not necessarily mean that there will be a high level of health or quality of life in a society. Even in some of the most affluent communities there are abundant social problems. The rich take advantage of the poor; the majority oppress the minority. Urbanization means loss of freedom as people begin to lose their identities and become cogs in the wheels of business and industry.

When people cease to regard each other as persons there is a loss of integrity which extends into business and politics. There is no longer equality of opportunity. People no longer trust each other. Justice is weighted on the side of the one who can pay.

If we are to have a healthy society we would do well
to remember Jesus' approach to the legalistic Pharisees
-- "you neglect the important things: justice, mercy,
and faith" (Matthew 23:23). The basic health worker
will find that the Bible provides the best advice that
can be given to a community for offering every member
dignity and a sense of meaning in life -- love your
neighbor as you love yourself (that is, with concern
for his welfare), and (in the same sense) love your
enemies as well.

Social health requires equity, justice, mercy,
discipline, freedom, and integrity, all permeated by
loving concern for each member. Prisons are filled
with people who need all of these. A healthy society
may well begin by developing programs of visiting,
rehabilitation, and re-employment of prisoners, not
because ex-offenders are better risks than non-
offenders, but bacause the community cares.

RELIGION AND HEALTH

From the beginning of recorded history human
societies have related religious feelings and practices
to the quest for health. According to William D.
Reyburn, in Cameroun

> . . . illness, the opposite of health . . .
> means poor health with accompanying poverty,
> lack of offspring, attacks of witchcraft,
> curses, and a long, hard run of just plain
> bad luck. People in such straits, and they
> are usually numerous, seek a religion whose
> purpose it is to restore health (Reyburn
> 1968:44).

The priest, shaman, medicine man, prophet or holy
man who healed has been found in nearly all societies.
In a commentary on the article by G. Morris Carstairs,
Medicine and Faith in Rural Rajasthan, Benjamin Paul
says:

> To the people of rural India . . . sickness is
> as much a moral as a physical crisis. In their
> conception the roots of illness extend into the

realm of human conduct and cosmic purpose. As a consequence they look for relief to ritual and reassurance, as well as to mundane medicines (Paul and Miller 1955:107).

The well-known cardiologist, Meyer Friedman, said on a television program that the loss of religious experience, ritual, and tradition is contributing to heart attacks and other health problems.

Why are these religious aspects so important to health? After investigating all schools of psycho-analysis, the psychiatrist James Mallory claims that human beings have three basic and very powerful psycho-logical needs -- to give and receive love; to know that there is an ultimate, transcendent purpose and meaning in life; and to know that they, the people, are of value. These are spiritual needs, and the health education teams need to be aware of them in order to teach basic health workers to integrate spiritual and physical healing into the lives of their people and communities. This requires an intimate knowledge of the religious forms and scriptures, how people worship and in what they put their faith.

Human beings are congenitally egocentric. Gradually we learn how disruptive and inappropriate egocentricity can be, and how undependable a basis for judging our own needs and seeking to meet them. Learning that we cannot trust ourselves leads to a feeling of insecurity. Either we try to suppress this feeling, or we must put our confidence in something or someone greater than ourselves.

Some people put their whole faith in fetishes or idols; some in social or national leaders; some in material wealth; some in a form of government, even fanatically as Nazism and Communism require. None of these, however, is dependable, and none gives value to the individual. Only the God whom Jesus Christ revealed combines a concern for each individual's well-being with a transcendent meaning and purpose in life.

The basic health worker will have to function as a counselor, replacing the pagan practices of shaman, medicine man, curando, or witch doctor with ways which

lead to what St. Paul called "the fruit of the Spirit."
This fruit begins to appear when an individual surren-
ders his innate egocentricity and puts his faith in
God and experiences a radical transformation (literally
a change at the very *root* of his being), a conversion.
He is no longer simply a part in the "carbon cycle,"
but *someone* who matters to God. St. Paul says that in
Christ we become new beings (II Corinthians 5:17).
People who have felt they were "less than nothing" now
feel they are "God's people" (I Peter 2:11).(31)

New spiritual values accompany physical and mental
well-being to produce a steadily improving quality of
life in the individual and in the community.(32) They
can be identified and measured by the resulting levels
of efficiency, integrity, concern for others, and
commitment to service, and by the number of innovations
for the common good.

ART IN TEACHING AND HEALING

In many societies the role of the basic health
worker in emphasizing spiritual values will not be
that of a preacher. Each culture has its special ways
of communicating the deepest feelings of its people.
Some of the most effective are art forms -- music,
dance, games, puppetry, drama, and the graphic arts.
One good way to communicate with many who cannot read
is through art. A good picture can be worth 10,000
words to the illiterate (Kjaerland 1973:362). It is
important to recognize, however, that not all art
forms are understood by all people. Here again it is
essential that materials be prepared by or under the
direction of one who knows the culture from the
inside. If stick figures or pictures drawn in perspective do not convey meaning, photographs of local
scenes showing problems and their solutions may be
the teaching method most likely to lead to change.

It is hard to overestimate the healing of mind,
emotions, body, "self," or soul that can be achieved
through the arts. We are thrilled and inspired by
Sibelius' *Finlandia*, Beethoven's *9th Symphony*,
Tchaikovsky's *1812 Overture*, Handel's *Messiah*, or
perhaps by a solo flute playing Indian or Chinese

music, but an African Zulu might not respond to these. Yet there is music and rhythm in every culture which can communicate the deepest human feelings or provide a tool for teaching almost any subject from scripture to family planning, from the multiplication tables to nutrition.

Each of the arts may have its own field for studying cultural forms, for example, ethnomusicology. Fables, proverbs, group interactions, and symbolic objects provide other indigenous learning modes and methods. (39) Health education teams can train basic health workers to use skills in certain art forms as exciting and valuable means of communicating effectively.

Communication is the key. The health education teams teach basic health workers in specific subjects. They also teach them where to go for information and what kinds of questions to ask, how to use what they learn, and how to teach others. This must be a continuous and expanding process of teaching and learning.

We will examine several existing community health programs to learn what makes them effective.

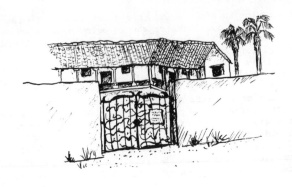

5

COMMUNITY HEALTH SERVICES
IN ACTION

The Goa border is only twenty miles south of Vengurla.
When Goa became part of India, we at St. Luke's
Hospital offered our services to the Goa Territory
Minister of Health. He told us that northern Goa,
nearest to us, was one of the areas most in need of
medical services, so we started a clinic there.

At first we worked one day a week in a small
Primary Health Center with the young government doctor
assigned there. The people had complained about
government medical services, especially the continual
rotation of doctors who refused to stay permanently in
such an isolated and poor part of Goa.

A wealthy local landowner, who had a building he
wanted to make into a hospital for the town, convinced
us that our services would be more valuable if we
moved our clinic from the center of town into more
spacious quarters which he would provide rent-free
about a mile away.

In the new location we were able to arrange the clinic to suit our convenience and to keep one of our own fully trained nurses there for case finding, continued treatments, and follow-up. We could even do operations there and make the clinic self-supporting. But all didn't go as we had hoped. The clinic is now closed.

There were several reasons for the clinic's failure. First, we left the center of town near the market place for a more isolated spot. The wealthy landowner was not a focus of influence among the people, but represented one of several factions. The nurse we assigned to the clinic was not from Goa, but from an entirely different culture and language area. We had started out working with and supplementing the government but ended by unintentionally duplicating many of its efforts. We failed to provide permanent up-to-date medical service to the people of northern Goa, not through lack of effort, but because the effort was misdirected.

Around the world many dedicated people are seeking more effective ways of extending health services to those who need them most, in rural areas and urban slums.(33) Here we present four examples of projects which emphasize training basic level health workers.

THE BEHRHORST-WORLD NEIGHBORS PROGRAM
CHIMALTENANGO, GUATEMALA

Carroll Behrhorst(34) began in 1962 a program that has pioneered in training a type of community basic health worker called a *promotor*. Behrhorst's unique and highly controversial project at Chimaltenango, Guatemala, was born out of a deep feeling of compassion for the local Indian population who so badly needed more health services.

The people needed simple curative medical care, more equitable land distribution, up-to-date agricultural methods, improved nutrution, better hygiene, and more adequate sanitation. Realizing that he could not deal with all of these needs alone, Behrhorst began to train

village leaders selected by local village priests,
Peace Corps workers, or himself.

The basic health workers are trained in two separate
groups meeting once a week at the Behrhorst Hospital
for three hours of classes and a period of bedside
clinical demonstration and teaching. This is much more
valuable to the students than formal lectures. Training is continuous. The rigorous curriculum includes:
treatment of a wide variety of common diseases diagnosed
by a review of symptoms rather than dependence on laboratory results; recognition of diseases that must be
referred to doctors immediately; sterile techniques;
emergency use of injections, especially for dehydration;
immunizations; use of the stethescope; methods for
improving nutrition, hygiene and sanitation; family
planning; and agricultural extension by soil sampling,
new seeds, and appropriate use of fertilizers.

A unique locally written manual is used to train
the rural paramedical workers, or promotors. The manual
names each disease; then the parts of the body affected
how the disease is transmitted, the diagnosis by signs
and symptoms, appropriate treatment or referral of the
patient, and methods of prevention are pictorially
described.(35)

After passing an examination following one year of
training, basic health workers may purchase medicines
at a concession rate from the hospital with low-interest
loans if necessary. Resale of these medicines by the
promotors to their patients provides part of the incentive for being in the program and helps to recoup
expenses for the time spent in training and in service.

There are a number of built-in ways of controlling
the quality of service rendered. One is through the
"Committee for Improvement" made up of the promotors
themselves who rotate on and off the committee every
four months. Another is requiring the turning in of
"patient forms" which must be filled out for each
patient treated. Only if these forms and informal
monthly examinations are satisfactorily completed will
the committee permit the promotor to purchase medicines. Still another control is the practive of having

the doctors in charge spend a day with two or three of the promotors at their own village "clinics."

Recently there has been a move for cooperation and control by the government public health services, no doubt motivated by the pioneering efforts of the Behrhorst program to do more village work.

From time to time additional projects have been aimed at teaching women in their homes or through women's clubs. Some of the topics studied are literacy, family planning, home gardens, poultry farms, animal husbandry, sewing and weaving, use of latrines, boiling of water and milk, keeping food covered and protected from flies, use of protein foods, dental hygiene, and prevention of the spread of tuberculosis.

In 1963 World Neighbors(36) began to support the agricultural training, self-help programs, and rotating loans to farmers for purchasing their own land.

Alan Greenwold, who joined the program in 1971, has special interest in opportunities for improved land tenure, employment, and housing. He has also been exploring the feasibility of selecting basic health workers through representative community health committees so that they may become instigators of community action and directors of public opinion. This borders on political action for rural development, possibly the most effective way of motivating a government to make appropriate improvements for a better quality of life for its citizens in rural areas.

INTEGRATED HEALTH SERVICES: PILOT STUDY PROJECT
MIRAJ, MAHARASHTRA STATE, INDIA

A new program based at the Miraj Medical Centre in Sangli District, Maharashtra, India, has complete government collaboration and support for seventy-seven workers assigned to it. This is the first time in India that so many government personnel have been placed under the authority of a church institution.

This project will serve a population of about 200,000 in fifty-two villages. In addition to

government funded staff, support comes from the United
Presbyterian Church, which has had a community health
and family planning program based at Miraj for over
ten years,(37) and from the Swedish International
Development Authority.

The director, Eric Ram, began the program with two
weeks of intensive orientation for trainers and super-
visory staff. This was followed by six weeks of
comprehensive training for Multipurpose Basic Health
workers and Integrated Auxiliary Nurse-Midwives(38) in
the philosophy, concept, scope, and details of integrated health services. The entire team includes 28
Multipurpose Basic Health Workers, 40 Auxiliary Nurse-
Midwives, 10 Health Visitor Nurse-Midwives, 2 Public
Health Nurses, 7 Integrated Health Inspectors, 2
Integrated Health Supervisors, and 1 Health Extension
Officer.

A Multipurpose Basic Health Worker, who serves
about 7,500 people, lives in a village and works out
of a Community Health Sub-Center housed in buildings
provided by village political leaders. His duties
are: (1) to gather all pertinent statistics; (2) to
report and help control or eradication of communicable
diseases such as tuberculosis, malaria, cholera,
typhoid, dysentery, hepatitis, smallpox, polio, and
leprosy; (3) to collect all necessary blood or sputum
specimens; (4) to assist with vaccinations and other
immunizations; (5) to conduct environmental sanitation
inspection; (6) to supervise building of latrines,
developing of water supplies, and proper drainage;
(7) to give instruction in family planning and nutrition; and (8) to assist in school health programs.

The Integrated Auxiliary Nurse-Midwife also lives
in a village, serves a population of 5,000, and is in
charge of the Community Health Sub-Center which is
visited weekly by a doctor. Her duties include: (1)
prenatal, natal, and postnatal care of mothers; (2)
referral of all abnormal cases to the appropriate
medical center; (3) infant and pre-school child care;
(4) family planning with an effort to reduce the
current birth rate by 10/1000 in five years; (5)
training of untrained village midwives; (6) routine
immunizations of infants, pre-school children, and

mothers; (7) health and nutrition education; (8) treatment of minor ailments; (9) follow-up on tuberculosis
and leprosy patients.

Health Inspectors supervise basic health workers,
organize mass surveys, and implement any necessary
remedial efforts.

The Health Supervisor coordinates the work of the
Health Inspectors and deals particularly with community
power structures for solving particular problems or
initiating new projects.

Government authorities are expected to subsidize the
whole program after three years if it is cost-effective
and can be duplicated in other parts of the state.

COMMUNITY HEALTH AND DEVELOPMENT PROJECT
KOJEDO, SOUTH KOREA

John Sibley directs the Kojedo Project on an island
six miles southeast of mainland Korea. The island is
twenty-one miles long and fifteen miles wide, with
only one qualified Western-trained doctor for its population of 120,000. The project was purposely located
on an isolated peninsula and has had to develop all
its own facilities and earn community cooperation.

As noted in *Contact 5* (Christian Medical Commission,
Oct., 1971), the Kojedo Project was developed to study
six possibilities: (1) a broad, community-centered
health program consisting of family planning, public
health, and a scientifically controlled, submaximal
curative medicine; (2) a coordinated community development effort to encourage the local residents to organize
and participate in cooperatives and other self-help
projects; (3) the program to be carried out in close
cooperation with and along the lines of the Korean
government's plans; (4) a major effort to adapt the
scope of the program to the potential resources of the
community, thus making self-support feasible; (5)
involving the church congregation at the village level
in the project as a concerned and motivating force;
and (6) avoiding major capital investments that cannot
be recovered or easily incorporated into other programs.

The following description of the project is quoted from *The Kojedo Project and Community Medicine* by permission of David Thurber, editor.

Staff: About twenty trained medical personnel including doctors, nurses, laboratory technicians, and nurse's aids employed.

Facilities: Small rural health center with twelve in-patient beds; delivery room; out-patient department; emergency room; operating room; maternal-child health and family planning, public health, health education, laboratory and X-ray facilities. Field experience in community health for medical students and student nurses is an active part of the program.

Motivation: The Christian concept of concern for "the least of these" makes it mandatory to consider the total health needs, physical, mental, and spiritual, of all people and try to find creative answers to the problems of uneven distribution of health services.

Purpose: To bring low-cost but comprehensive health care to a defined population of a rural area, with the expectation that its successful elements might be incorporated in that aspect of national planning having to do with rural health systems.

Project Functions:

I. Direct Service Aspect (in school, village, church, clinic)

   A. Programs

      1. Out-patient clinic
      2. In-patient care
      3. Public health
      4. Maternal and child health and family planning
      5. School health

6. Resident village aide and regional nurse service
7. Village volunteer service
8. Patient follow-up service
9. Druggist education
10. Sunday school

B. Activities

1. Health education

   a. family planning
   b. child health
   c. maternal health
   d. dental health
   e. tuberculosis
   f. sanitation
   g. evangelism
   h. agriculture

2. Preventive care

   a. well-baby care and immunizations
   b. prenatal and postnatal care
   c. family planning
   d. dental care
   e. village water supply
   f. agriculture

3. Simple curative care

   a. medical
   b. surgical
   c. obstetrical
   d. dental

II. Broader Educational Aspect (not the responsibility of a 100 percent service-oriented project)

1. Evaluation and Planning
2. Resident Training
3. Medical Student Training
4. Nursing Student Training
5. Army-Police Medic Training

       6. In-service Training
           a. regional nurse
           b. clinic aides
           c. village aides
           d. clinical sociological conference
       7. Druggist Training
       8. School Teacher Training
       9. Medical Insurance Development
      10. Statistical Reports

The project has become primarily a community medica
care teaching institution, as the need for strong
emphasis on education at all levels has become evi-
dent. Two forms of education can be distinguished.
First is the education that is a fundamental requisite
of the ongoing service aspects of the project, a many-
pronged teaching program aimed at the whole community
and carried out by staff personnel at the project
center and in villages . . . . Public health teaching
activities include school education; child care clinic
at the project; church group education; teaching
mothers' clubs, 4-H clubs, and other village groups;
and single or group discussions with patients at the
clinic and with villagers when the public health team
goes to a village for immunizations and patient follow
up visiting . . . .

The other form of education is designed for a wider
audience: staff of the project, medical professionals
and others concerned with the development of effective
forms of medical care within Korea and without . . . .

The paramedical worker, or medical auxiliary, is an
individual trained to carry out specifically defined
activities . . . essential in a health delivery system
. . . which do not require the advanced training of a
physician or nurse. The doctor and nurse, thus freed
for concentration on the more technical aspects of
health care, are enabled to . . . increase the scope
of their activities, both quantitatively and qualita-
tively. It is required of the physician, however,
(1) that he clearly define those areas of care deliver
that paramedical personnel can satisfactorily cover,
(2) that he provide for adequate training of the worke
to carry out those duties, and (3) that he provide for
continued training and supervision . . . .

The Kojedo Project has been experimenting with a number of ways of using paramedical workers. This has been made more difficult by Korea's strict medical-legal codes -- similar to codes that existed in much of the United States before recent changes in many states allowing the use of supervised paramedical personnel -- that prohibit treatment by anyone other than a licensed physician.

The effectiveness of a community health program will be directly proportional to the degree to which it can sustain an active, stimulating influence for health in every home in each individual village. Where health gaps are large, this sustained influence can best be maintained, not by occasional visits of a health team, but only by the constant physical presence in the village of a trained representative of that team, a paramedical worker . . . .

Developing health in an area that has had no under-standing of it takes more than occasional education, maternal and child care, and an immunization program. The project, in the spring of 1973, started an experi-mental program of nurse aides living in four villages that had previously had no near source of health care at all. Their role is to supply two parts of the pyramid of a graduated health system -- first to con-stantly work at developing a base of knowledge of health principles so that it becomes a part of every-one's life, from a mother taking care to keep flies away from the food she is preparing, and a father covering his cough, to a farmer not using raw night-soil on his fields; and second to fill the long-term need in a graduated system for someone to give simple primary prenatal, child, adolescent, and adult care, controlled by a doctor through strict standing-order direction, and to refer those who need more advanced care to a nurse or a doctor. It is hoped that the nurse aide, by living in a village for an extended period of time, will have a considerable ability to educate -- by talking to people as friends, by point-ing out bad techniques, by being an example to others, in addition to frequent teaching in the local school and to various groups; and that by having a full-time member teaching health the village will become con-scious of health full-time. Medical treatment by

anyone other than a doctor or senior medical student
remains illegal in Korea, and the project is still
trying to gain more than implicit official approval
for the program.

Several members of the project staff visited a
number of villages to propose to leaders the idea of
the village aide program. All the villages were enthu-
siastic about having someone who could give medical
treatment; but instead of the idea of health care bein
a commodity that is available for purchase, the projec
wanted to encourage a feeling of common responsibility
for the development of health. Each village was asked
if it would be interested in setting up a village
health committee that would make all the basic decisions and arrangements for health care in the village
-- providing a place for the aide to live and treat,
planning health education and a preventive health
program with the aide and regional nurse, and deciding
rates for treatment with the eventual goal of paying
the aide's full salary. This is quite a different way
of looking at medical care, and some people responded
more strongly than others. A high level of interest
was the most important criterion used in deciding
where the aides would go . . . .

Local Christian Involvement:

We must be particularly aware of human values when
a doctor needs to see a large number of patients a
day. A well-loved deaconess in a local church is
available full-time in the clinic waiting room, showing concern, finding out information about patients
that a doctor is not likely to discover, serving tea,
being patient advocate when someone is not satisfied
with the care he is receiving, and sharing her Christian beliefs with those who are interested . . . .

Once a week the minister of the nearest church
leads the morning staff chapel service. Close ties
have developed between his church and the project.
Because a number of church members are either on the
project's staff or on the board of directors, the
congregation has been able to feel closely involved
in caring for others, an involvement which has
increased because of the minister's strong leadership

in . . . understanding . . . the active responsibility
of all of us for each other . . . .

- - - - -

The Kojedo Project has had an uphill struggle for
recognition and cooperation by medical schools, government health authorities, and local practitioners. Since
the writing of the above report the central government
has not only given favorable notice to the project, but
also asked that it greatly expand its facilities. The
government has also offered to subsidize and help
expand the project's community health insurance plan
so that it may become a model for the rest of South
Korea.

COMPREHENSIVE RURAL HEALTH PROJECT
JAMKHED, MAHARASHTRA STATE, INDIA

(Condenses from a longer report by R. S. Arole
published in *Contact 10*(39), August 1972, and quoted
by permission of James McGilvray, Director, Christian
Medical Commission, World Council of Churches. Drs.
Rajanikant and Mabelle Arole, both graduates of the
Christian Medical College, Vellore, India, direct this
project. Their initial planning played a significant
part in the project's success.)

Since the problems in rural areas relating to health
are many, we set the following priorities:

1. to make available facilities and personnel in
   rural areas;

2. to do something about the rapid population
   explosion;

3. to attempt to reduce the high infant mortality
   and continued mortality and morbidity up to
   the age of five;

4. to take care of certain chronic diseases which
   not only contribute to mortality but also morbidity in the society and which, more than that,
   deprive the people of their dignity, especially
   those suffering from leprosy.

The goal was to develop a program which would be
fitted to the needs of the community but which would
also be compatible with the resources available to the
community.

The method was to establish a main center in the
central area, i.e., at Jamkhed, where we would have
diagnostic help, facilities for emergency surgery and
emergency medical care. There would be ten sub-centers
in ten surrounding villages, the maximum distance
between the central village and the sub-centers being
ten miles. For this program we would need to use
auxiliary workers and paramedical workers; we would
need the cooperation and involvement of the indigenous
practitioners, other health officials, school teachers,
and dais (indigenous midwives). There was to be
cooperation with . . . government programs. And
finally at the end of six years this would have to be
a self-supporting program. For a program to be self-
supporting, motivation would have to be developed in
the community and the community leaders, the local,
state, and the central government taking responsibility
for this kind of work.

Objectives

1. Reduce birthrate from 40/1000 to 30/1000

2. Reduce under fives' mortality by 50%

3. Identify and bring under regular treatment
    leprosy and tuberculosis patients.

4. Train indigenous workers and offer field
    training to health workers.

. . . we decided that we would go to an area where
there was no Christian witness because we wanted to
establish a Christian witness in an entirely non-
Christian area. Secondly, we wanted an area where
there was an acute need for medical care and where
there was no [other likelihood] of any future development . . . . This area, like many other rural areas
of India, has a very strong caste system. About 50
percent of the people are cultivators or farmers: 20
percent are untouchables -- the people who are very

poor and usually landless laborers -- who socially have
no status.

The villages have a governing board with an elected
head called the Sarpanch . . . . One cannot enter any
community by bypassing the leaders, because if a leader
feels that he has not been given due recognition, he
can become hostile and uncooperative.

We said, "If you want us to come into your area,
there are certain things that you should be prepared
to do. We shall be about twenty to twenty-five health
workers coming into your area without having any housing facilities. We expect you to make some arrangements for accommodation for about twenty people . . . [and]
temporary buildings for our clinics and our diagnostic
facilities, and if after a six-month period we find
that your interest in us remains, you should donate us
land to build permanent structures in your area."

. . . we laid conditions under which we would be
willing to go to the area, and they were willing to
fulfill these conditions. They emptied out an old
veterinary dispensary, about 30 x 10 feet, which we
used as our out-patient department. They gave us a
storage place for in-patients and rented a place for
us to live. It was a very simple arrangement -- no
electricity, no running water, and all twenty of us
having to live in a 20 x 30 foot area.

We formed a consultative committee which consisted
of not only members of this local village but others
from different areas, representing different communities, especially the poor "harijan" (untouchable)
community. The first responsibility we gave this
committee was to find accommodation for us and accommodation for our health center. We then asked them to
find us staff. Most of our staff, like nurses and
paramedical workers, had to be brought from the city.
This staff had to be Christian because we were there
to establish a Christian witness and at the same time
give medical care . . . .

Besides this nucleus of Christian staff we needed
other people -- the non-professionals from the community. We asked our consultative committee to hire these

for us. This had an advantage as they wanted to do
their best for us, for we had told them that if within
six months we did not have a good response from them,
we would find some other place to work . . . .

After that we went around from village to village,
holding meetings in each village. Our first objective
was to get an idea of the felt needs . . . . We dis-
cussed with the members of the community our interest
to improve their health, but they felt that curative
care should take precedence over other programs that
we were proposing to them. We told them if they were
willing to pay for these services, we would start with
these. They all agreed to this; so from the first day
we have been self-supporting as far as the curative
work is concerned . . . .

As the news spread to the nearby villages, people
became aware that they could come and negotiate with
us to go to their villages. Here again we said, "The
decision to start work in your village area is entirely
up to you. These are our conditions: If you want us
to come . . . to start health work, you give us a place
to work, give us your cooperation, give us your help
in child care and immunization of your children, give
full cooperation to our team, and care for our nurses
when they stay in your villages . . . .

We are located at the border of three counties. If
we were in one county, the political leaders would
probably feel that they could put pressure on us; but
lcoated as we are, we can move from one county to
another to avoid such pressures. We asked one of the
local men how we could get away if we did not get the
required cooperation within six months. He suggested
that we build a center using tin sheets as a shed
. . . . The entire building can be dismantled and
reconstructed within fifteen days by the firm which
built it.

I would like to describe a typical encounter with a
village. We usually go in the evening because that is
the time when the villager is relaxed, and we go and
call the village leaders. The leaders feel important
that a doctor has left his place and come all the way
to their village. We are usually given tea, and we

start our discussion. Very often we find that the uppermost thing in their minds, even when talking to a doctor, is not health; the usual question is food. This was especially so because there was a famine when we entered the area. We take their lead and discuss food for the children. Then we go into the topic of malnutrition, and we . . . say, "Your children do not have enough food. Maybe we can get some agency involved and interested in getting some milk for your children. What will you do in return?" And the villagers . . . come up with the idea that they will bring some things from their own homes and make a common meal for the children. Those who are able will donate some money, and those who have no money will contribute labor.

So right then and there we form a committee . . . responsible for cooking the food. The responsibility means purchasing fuel and utensils, maintaining daily records, and getting the children together for the meal. This committee then appoints people who will collect the money for the fuel and utensils and takes charge of the feeding program . . . . We did not impose this program on them. We went and talked about their felt need, and the felt need was food, and gradually we translated that into a supplementary feeding program for children under five . . . .

We realized that the second most needed item is water for farming and drinking. So we put another proposal to the villagers . . . "Your children are being fed . . . now, but this is not going to be permanent. Why don't we think of something else which will be more permanent . . .?" We propose making wells . . . .

So the committee decides to find a permanent solution for the undernourished children in the village by getting a well sunk. Then we translate this community action into a scientific action. There are agencies in that area which are working with boring machines for water supply and sinking wells. We get this team to come and do a survey [and decide on the most likely places to strike water]. To date there are ten wells where we have struck water, and six of these wells have enough water for irrigation. So after this monsoon we shall have fifteen acres of land to grow

rich protein food. Now we are sure that when this
experience works, there will be more farmers who will
be interested and will make land available for feeding
children of the entire village. So again we helped
the community to decide just by encouraging them and
helping them to arrive at the decision . . . .

We do not always go and listen to the problems of
the villagers. Sometimes we sit with the village people
and talk to them about our problems -- for example, the
problem of getting to their villages because the roads
are so bad -- and if they really want us to come to
their villages, what can they do? Already the villagers
have made a seven-mile road connecting two centers; the
minister has had fifty miles of road paved to the
villages. Making the roads or paving the roads is not
important, but what is important is that the people
wanted us and the care we could offer them so that they
were willing to pay for the care and share the responsibility for it as well . . . .

Children are immunized at the center. Immunization
is only done in the villages when the villagers fulfill
certain conditions . . . namely . . . collect at least
80 percent of the children, list their names, weigh
them, and then send us word to come to inoculate them.
When we arrive at the village, we get the school
teacher or the Sarpanch to tell the people the reason
for our being there and what to expect as possible
reactions from the immunizations given. We usually
give some drugs such as aspirins to the Sarpanch, and
he tells his people that if they should have any
reactions, he will give them medicines.

In school health the school teachers take a major
part. They list the children, test their sight,
weigh them and help us during their examinations. We
leave with them drugs for treatment that may be
required . . . .

We do not have separate clinics for leprosy patients.
We do not go to the leprosy patients' homes; they all
come to the center . . . .

Our survey work is done by a team, not by one person
alone. Usually in the team there is a nurse, an

auxiliary nurse-midwife, a special family planning
worker, a basic health worker and a laboratory technician. The team goes from house to house. Nobody
knows who is looking for a leprosy patch. The team
surveys a family for antenatal patients, for children
under five, for patients with a chronic cough, and for
those with a skin lesion. So child care, antenatal
care, treatment for leprosy and tuberculosis can be
given. The nurses are supplied with simple drugs
. . . .

In rural work due respect has to be given to the
indigenous practitioner. These indigenous practitioners are usually rebuffed by trained doctors. We are
naturally a threat to them. So we have established a
rapport with them, taken steps to ensure their friendship, making sure not to bypass them or belittle them.
We seek their cooperation in feeding programs for
children, treatment of leprosy and tuberculosis. We
give them drugs and so involve them in the treatment
of village patients. We also explain . . . the important role their wives can play in the care of
antenatal cases. Two wives of indigenous practitioners are already attending the hospital for help towards
giving such services. During the school vacation we
are involving the school children in areas of nutrition, sanitation, and family planning. We have found
these youth groups can play an active part, particularly
in family planning.

The Jamkhed Rural Health Project started by locating
an area where a population of 80,000 lacked medical
care and where the villages were within ten miles of
the central emergency care hospital. It depended
heavily on community cooperation from the beginning.

- - - - -

HOLDING FAST TO WHAT IS GOOD

Two of the four programs outlined here are included
in *Health by the People*, published by the World Health
Organization in Geneva in 1975. The editor, Kenneth W.
Newell, Director, Division of Strengthening Health
Services, WHO, comments that the success of a variety
of attempts to solve problems shows clearly that some

of the questions do have answers, and there is no need
for the world to wait for some single universal
answer. "The trail blazers," he says, "have been out
ahead . . . . The 'optimal solution,' if such a thing
ever existed, is not here but progressive courses of
action towards an acceptable solution are with us.

Certain characteristics of one or more of the projects seem to us particularly important:

1. A basic motivation, arising from a commitment
   to Jesus Christ, to serve those having the
   greatest need -- principally the poor, and often
   the despised.

2. Locating and working in the place where the
   greatest number of those in need live.

3. A team approach to continuous non-formal in-
   service training and supervision of multipurpose
   basic health workers, especially those who are
   already serving as indigenous practitioners.

4. Use of highly motivated volunteers whose service
   gives them a sense of self-worth.

5. An integrated, holistic approach to health services including literacy, water supply, farm
   loans, and agriculture extension programs
   whenever possible.

6. Emphasis on setting objectives such as reducing
   high infant mortality and malnutrition.

7. Concentration on public health and family
   planning.

8. Obtaining cooperation of acknowledged local
   power structures for these and additional
   development programs.

9. Follow-up on patients who are cured or under
   treatment.

10. Use of an established base capable of self-
    support, or development of such a base, for a
    health extension program.

11. Using curative services to give credibility and support to preventive medical and public health programs.

12. Experiments with ways to make the programs self-supporting, cost-effective, and continuous so that they can be duplicated.

13. Efforts to obtain recognition, cooperation, and support from national governments.

None of the four model projects is completely self-supporting. Some others are (Nugroho, 1972). None of the four has yet fully integrated all available resources to improve the health of its community. Some have approached this goal.(40) All four projects now enjoy local community approval and national government recognition -- encouraging steps toward permanent health extension.

We have used the above characteristics and goals in designing a model for fully integrated training in community health services which can be adjusted as necessary to fit local circumstances.

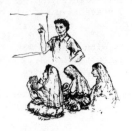

6

A MODEL PROGRAM FOR
HEALTH EDUCATION BY EXTENSION

In addition to all the usual functions of a 150-bed
mission hospital -- general medicine, general and
specialized surgery, obstetrics, gynecology, and pedi-
atrics for in-patients; general practice in the out-
patient department; administration; and evangelism --
we set up a community health service. No one was
assigned exclusively to this serive. It was everyone's
business.

One of our male nurses taught first aid in the
schools and to the church women's group. The doctors
conducted annual physical examinations in the schools
and prescribed treatment as required. Student nurses,
assisted by college students, conducted community
health surveys. Our public health-family planning
nurse worked with government supported auxiliary
nurse-midwives in their own villages. We expanded our
immunization program to include smallpox, B.C.G., and
polio vaccination and triple antigen. In villages and
in our hospital out-patient department we distributed
literature on the prevention and treatment of intestinal
parasites, scabies, and tuberculosis and on proper care

of infants and mothers. We started free under-fives, maternity, and tuberculosis clinics at the hospital.

With the Indian government putting more and more stress on the importance of family planning we devised a vaginal tubectomy operation which became so popular that our hospital team was in constant demand to perform this type of tubal ligation in government arranged family planning "camps" throughout the district. Our strength and our supplies were often exhausted as we completed up to 100 operations a day. In spite of the fact that we worked in small primary health centers without screens or running water we had no complications. The results were gratifying and profitable both to the patients and to the hospital.

We held a number of meetings with village leaders in the area around Vengurla, asking what they felt were their greatest needs. Invariably they were for health services. Everyone wanted us to start our own mobile health clinics again. We told them we would do better -- we would work with registered medical practitioners (homeopathic, ayurvedic, and others) who were already practicing in or near the villages. These were our basic health workers. We consulted with these practitioners on their difficult cases. We arranged for visiting specialists to conduct classes at our hospital to update the training of the local practitioners, and we provided them with certain allopathic drugs and tried to teach them by non-formal in-service instruction how best to use these medicines.

This kind of training requires the utmost tact, patience, and sincerity, but we hope it will result in improved village health care. We met one objection -- a realistic one -- that our free consultations and teaching periods caused the local practitioners some loss of time and income. The latter might have been remedied by charging fees, but we did not do so because we wanted to test this factor on a limited basis.

Finally we talked with the village leaders about revolving loans available to their local farmers and how their communities could benefit from food-for-work programs. There are still many other things which can be done for community improvement.

In his book, *Out of the African Night*, William
Reyburn points out that "health" to the African includes
what we in the West would call

> . . . bodily health, emotional stability, finan-
> cial security, freedom from fear and anxiety,
> all-round good luck, and a batch of healthy off-
> spring. This may sound like far too many good
> things to roll up in the word "health," but many
> African peoples see all of these blessings
> accruing in a natural way to the person who is
> *whole* (Reyburn 1968).

It is exactly this health for the whole person which we
hope to achieve through the use of basic health workers
trained by in-service extension education. The plan
presented here can be adapted to the particular needs
of each local community.

A DESIGN FOR
COORDINATED COMMUNITY HEALTH SERVICES

Area Health Service Teams will be formed in conjunction with a local hospital, clinic, college, seminary,
or other self-supporting base and will be composed of
doctors, nurses, paramedics, school teachers, social
workers, agriculturists, nutritionists, pastors, and
others who are needed and available.

Surveys

The Area Health Service Teams, assisted by school
teachers, students, and other volunteers will carry
out surveys of carefully defined and properly sampled
communities, studying the following health parameters:

a. Age and sex, birth rates, births by age/parity
    of mother, rates of population growth.

b. Patterns of migration; occupation/education of
    parents.

c. Infant death rates, maternal death rates, suicid
    rates, weight by age of children under five year
    old, family providers' disability days/year.

d. Most prevalent and serious diseases at specific ages.

e. Most frequent causes of death and disability.

f. Environmental and agricultural needs of the communities.

g. Current spending by people on all forms of health services.

h. Health (medical, agricultural, educational, industrial, financial, cultural, and spiritual) resources -- available and potential, indigenous and non-indigenous.

i. Rates of utilization of health services (clinic visits, hospital beds, and other facilities) by various segments of the population.

j. Patterns of community organization.

k. Local educational, cultural, and religious patterns that relate to health, and use of all community development services.

Program Design

On the basis of survey results, together with locally derived understanding, the Area Health Service Teams will (1) assign priorities among the health and economic problems, using such criteria as prevalence, seriousness, vulnerability to management, and community concern; (2) assess the possibilities of coordinating all resources (government, secular, voluntary, etc.) in the development of health programs; and (3) design and implement programs whose goals are to provide maximum improvement with the least cost in those health areas which have been assigned highest priority.

Dr. John Bryant has developed a useful method of determining priorities among objectives (Bryant 1970: 75). It begins with a survey conducted by advocates and innovators to discover the local health problems. Each of the problems is then given a rating from 0 to 4 under each of the following headings: prevalence,

seriousness, community concern, and vulnerability to
management. Finally, all the points for each health
problem are multiplied. The score for any problem
determines its priority among the objectives. This
formula is also applicable to problems other than
medical or public health. According to Fred Sai,

> The weight put on any one of [the criteria for
> granting priorities] will depend on local cir-
> cumstances and how a particular program can have
> a multiplying effort or hold the key to others
> (Sai 1973).

The priority list will be re-evaluated from time to
time.

Although priorities may differ in each community,
as will forms of training, a typical program will start
with the development of Training Teams by the Area
Health Service Teams. The Training Teams may include
existing hospital, clinic, or other institutional
staff having different skills, who will in turn teach
men and women selected by their own local communities
to be Basic Health Workers.(41) An essential part of
the program is continuous in-service extension education, encouragement, and supervision of these Basic
Health Workers as they serve in their own communities.
This will be done by the Training Teams through one or
more of the following plans:

1. Weekly at the base institution with trainees
   attending lectures, rounds, and demonstrations.

2. Weekly in the Basic Health Workers' communities
   or villages by on-the-job in-service training.

3. One or two weeks of intensive training at the
   base institution twice a year alternating with
   supervised community or village service.

The Training Teams have the primary responsibility
of teaching the Basic Health Workers health care and
its promotion and other ways of improving the quality
of life. The teams, attached to the base institutions
which will be referral centers for the program, will
teach and supervise a minimum of five Basic Health

Workers annually, a total of twenty-five over five years. Each Basic Health worker will serve a maximum community population of 2,500. Thus the program is designed to serve as many as 62,500 people by the end of five years.

Basic Health Workers may earn their livelihood or derive other forms of satisfaction from their health training. Each Basic Health Worker will have the back-up support of and be responsible to a local Community Development Committee for primary health care and health teaching. Together they will plan for health facilities, the delivery of coordinated community health services, and additional development programs. (See Appendix B)

Program Objectives

Each program will be built around specific objectives determined by the area survey, but all should lead to attainment of the following general goals as coordinated community health services become established through trained Basic Health Workers:

1. Decrease in infant death rates.

2. Decrease in maternal death rates.

3. Improvement in nutritional status of children under the age of five years.

4. Decrease in the family providers' average number of disability days/year.

5. Decrease in birth rates and increase in birth intervals by family planning where this is appropriate to the situation.

6. Decrease in most serious and prevalent diseases when these are vulnerable to management.

7. Increase in the number of people having access to all health services.

8. Improvements in the economic level of each family.

9. Increase in utilization of all community
    development projects.

10. Dynamic integration of all of human life.

Field Director

A Field Director will direct the program. After
surveys have been completed, the Director will advise
on the methods of health planning, community development, locating potential Basic Health Workers, and
instructing the Training Teams. The Director will
research, develop, and recommend manuals, correspon-
dence courses, audiovisuals, and other teaching aids
in order to continually update and assist Training
Teams to be more effective.(42) Without being a participant, the Field Director will coordinate the
periodic and final evaluation of the whole program
which will include the performance of his/her own role
and responsibilities.

Evaluation

Continuous evaluation of the program in each of its
locations will be made by an "in-house" committee or
team as well as by a third party -- for example,
central governments, foundations, or the World Health
Organization -- after the first, third, and fifth
years.

Surveys made at the beginning of the program by
Area Health Service Teams will be repeated for measur-
ing achievement of program objectives and making
regenerative or formative evaluations for mid-course
corrections. Most of the re-surveys will be done by
those teams plus the Basic Health Workers and Training
Teams, with the final evaluations made by the third
party.

In consultation with the health Training Teams,
Basic Health Workers, and local community development
committees, the Area Health Service Teams will
redesignate priorities as necessary.

The possibilities of further integrating all health
resources will be reassessed and recommendations made
in the same consultation.

Recommendations will be made on the kinds of health promoting services which communities are able and willing to support with gradual reduction of outside support for various programs that have demonstrated their cost-effectiveness.

Recommendations for interim modifications of each project or the total program will be made at the end of the first and third years.

After the fifth year, final evaluation and assessment of each project, and an overview and evaluation of the entire program will be made by the third party, with publication of pertinent findings and recommendations made, again in consultation with the local community development committees, the Basic Health Workers, the Training Teams, and the Area Health Service Teams. That evaluation will indicate to what extent the purpose and objectives of the program have been fulfilled, and will suggest specific recommendations about the use of such models in other situations.

It is deceptively simplistic to try to draw up a design for perfecting any community or society without taking into account gross differences between cultures and constant problems caused by egocentric human nature. In fact, if mankind could become transformed -- converted -- into people who really cared about each other, it might not be necessary to design such programs at all. As one pastor told his church officers, more healing is achieved through love than in any other way.(43) Where does this healing love come from?

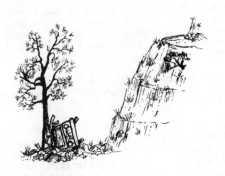

7

THE MESSENGERS AND THE MESSAGE

It was ten o'clock on a Saturday night when the police called. There had been an accident on the road near Kankavli, thirty-five miles away. Would I take a team from the hospital and go there?

As soon as we could gather splints, bandages, and other first aid supplies, four of us started off in the ambulance, but it was midnight before we arrived at Kankavli.

The police had not said what kind of accident, and we were totally unprepared for what we found. On the porch of the local primary health center were fifty dead. Inside on the floor were more than fifty injured -- many in shock, most with fractures, some with multiple compound fractures and other injuries.

An open truck carrying more than 100 men and boys to a singing competition had failed to negotiate a curve and had rolled down an embankment. We were the first medical team to arrive, but the police had already moved all of the victims -- unsplinted -- from the scene of the accident to the primary health center

We did what we could, applying splints, starting intravenous solutions, dressing wounds, and trying to encourage the injured and their frightened relatives and friends. There was little comfort we could give the relatives of the dead and dying.

The police commandeered another large truck to take the most seriously injured to St. Luke's Hospital and a bus to take others to the government hospital twenty miles away.

In Vengurla the hospital staff had prepared several beds, expecting victims of an automobile accident. When forty seriously injured patients arrived at our 100-bed hospital about 4:30 A.M. the nurses and attendants quickly moved convalescing patients to mattresses on the floor of the out-patient department to make room in the wards and on verandahs for the new arrivals.

By 6 A.M. we had returned with a few more injured in the ambulance. The off-duty staff members from doctors and nurses to sweepers had joined those on night duty, and no one left. One by one the patients were assigned to beds, taken for X-rays, and sent to the plaster room. The X-ray and laboratory technician was one of the team who had gone to the accident scene. He began to take X-rays as soon as we returned and took more than 100 before joining his colleague in the lab matching blood for those who needed transfusions.

Town officials arrived, and district officials, and state officials. Relatives of the injured and curious townspeople packed the verandahs and passages and milled around outside. In the church across the street the shaken congregation, much depleted by the absence of hospital staff members, prayed for the injured by name.

The staff worked on. The doctors operated on those with the most serious injuries. Wives and neighbors kept ice water, thermos bottles of hot tea, and tins of cookies just outside the operating room for staff members who did not leave even to eat.

It was 10 P.M. Sunday when the last surgical patient was lifted from the stretcher to a ward bed,

and the last cast was applied. Some of the staff had
had no rest for thirty-six hours; many had been working
for twenty-four. Their dedication and compassion,
their concern for the patients had done as much as
their medical skill to relieve the suffering of the
injured and terrified.

In a few days the patients we had sent to the government hospital began to arrive at St. Luke's. They had
heard that at the mission hospital there was something
more than medical treatment -- there they really cared
about you.

When the Chief Minister of Maharashtra State spoke
at the hospital's Fiftieth Anniversary celebration of
the need for everyone to exhibit more of the "missionary spirit," he was referring to the kind of selfless
caring for others that patients and their relatives
have seen demonstrated by the staff of St. Luke's
Hospital.

WHO CAN'T AND WHO CAN

Of all the groups into which the people of the
world are divided -- geographical, political, linguis-
tic, religious -- at this time only two are universal
enough and sufficiently motivated to transform society
in order to make health possible for the world. These
are the Communists and the Christians.

Marx said that religion is the opiate of the people
He claimed to be an atheist, and strangely, through
the influence of theologians Strauss and Bauer and the
French philosopher Feuerbach, (44) he became a militant
materialist. But in a heroic effort to perfect the
world without the help of the world's Creator Marx's
followers, the Communists, have built up a new system
of faith -- a religion of the "non-god" state. They
have their own master, circle of disciples, community
of professional followers, traditions, canon, doctrine
confession, recitations, rituals, symbols, and holiday
This religion has become the opiate of nearly one-thir
of the world's people.

In an effort to enforce complete equality in a classless society, Communism has stifled initiative. It has thus disqualified itself for offering health in a holistic sense. While it can develop medical and public health programs that will be attractive to people in great need, the "religion" of enforced conformity does not permit the celebration of each person's uniqueness; it does not enable achievement of the maximum potential in each person, that is, health.

Nor can individualistic Western secularism promote worldwide health. The idea that man is what he makes of himself, that he must pull himself up by his own bootstraps, leads to a lack of concern or even to contempt for the less fortunate. We are seeing in Western secular societies the deadly indifference and the spiritual emptiness that results when man sees himself as the center of the universe, when he devotes all his energies to achieving "the good life" for himself. Secularism is natural egocentricity on a massive scale, as disruptive and inappropriate to society as that of the infant to its family. Without discipline, cooperation, or integrity it cannot offer hope or help for the health of the world.

The New Testament tells us quite plainly what happens when human nature is left without the integrating, coordinating effort of a Christian world view:

> What human nature does is quite plain. It shows itself in immoral, filthy, and indecent actions . . . . People become enemies, they fight, become jealous, angry and ambitious . . . they are envious, get drunk, have orgies and do other things like these (Galatians 5:19-21, TEV).

Our daily newspapers confirm that this is indeed the case.

Human nature is selfish, self-centered, and eventually, self-destructive. It is the natural self-centeredness of man that has caused so many of the world's problems and prevented their solution. Dean Arthur F. Glasser of the Fuller Theological Seminary

School of World Mission reminds us that we are not
self-made:

> Man's dignity is derived from and dependent upon
> a right relationship to God, his Creator and
> Redeemer . . . .
>
> Man's relation to his fellowman depends upon
> his sense of personal accountability to God. If
> accountable only to another man, he eventually
> loses his personal freedom. One's accounta-
> bility to God involves commitment to love his
> fellowman.
>
> Man's service to God by honest and fearless
> thinking is essential to his experiencing of
> God's love for him and through him to others.
> If man fails to develop and use to the full
> his God-given capacities and talents [our
> ultimate criterion of health], he is failing
> in the dimension of love by limiting his use-
> fulness to his fellowman (Glasser 15).

The Christian's motivation thus comes from a
different source. His chief aim is not to perfect
society but to serve God. Since "the God of Scripture
does not limit his interest to so-called 'spiritual
things' but is concerned with the totality of the
world's life" (Smart) we find God's people -- that
is, the Christian Church -- uniquely qualified to
pioneer in developing worldwide holistic health
programs.

THE HEALTH-SALVATION RELATIONSHIP

Luke, who wrote the most extensive records we have
of Jesus' healing ministry, was a Greek physician.
The introduction to his book, *The Gospel of Luke*,
shows that he "was conscious that he was engaged upon
a task of vast historical importance. He dedicated
to it all he had -- a polished style, diligence, and
a careful, ordered mind" (Blaiklock 1968:3). We can
assume then that his words, written in his mother
tongue, were not chosen haphazardly, but to convey
precisely the facts as he saw them.

A woman who had been bleeding for twelve years was healed when she touched Jesus' clothes. When she confessed that she had done so, Luke tells us, Jesus said to the woman, "Daughter, your faith has made you well" (Luke 8:48, RSV). The word he used is *sodzo* (heal, cure, make well, make whole, save from sickness and suffering) -- physically healed.

Again in the story of the demon-possessed man from the Gergesene country, Luke records that when the people saw the former paranoid-schizophrenic sitting at Jesus' feet "clothed and in his right mind . . . the spectators told them how the madman had been cured" (*sodzo*) -- mentally healed (Luke 8:26-39, NEB).

Luke also describes the radical transformation in a tax collector named Zacchaeus that resulted from his encounter with Jesus (Luke 19:1-10, RSV). That Zacchaeus had been transformed -- converted -- is plain from his words: "Behold, Lord, the half of my goods I give to the poor, and if I have defrauded anyone of anything, I restore it fourfold." Jesus answered, "Today salvation has come to this house . . . . For the Son of Man came to seek and to save the lost." The word for "save" is again *sodzo* -- spiritual and social healing -- for a right relationship to God had transformed Zacchaeus' relationship to men.

Since Greek philosophy saw human beings as divided into mind, body, and spirit, it is remarkable that Luke saw healing in these different contexts as the same process. Health as Luke saw it was wholeness of mind, body, and spirit. This to him was salvation. We learn from Luke that a person's "soul," a word better translated "self," cannot be properly or fully saved apart from his being saved as a whole -- physically, mentally, emotionally, socially, and spiritually.

From a Hebrew point of view -- Jesus' own -- there was nothing unusual in viewing man as a unity. Jesus' concept of mankind is expressed by the Hebrew word *nephesh*, which is

. . . *the essential being of man*. It is the seat of man's emotions, feelings, passions, selfhood, desire, and life. Flesh and soul

are integral terms of a common being . . . .
Nephesh is commonly understood in relationship
to a physically identifiable structure of the
human being . . . which is man's total being,
his essential self, his living soul . . . .
There is no body/soul dualism in Hebrew
(Anderson).

Healing those who were physically ill was to Jesus
neither more nor less important than discussing theology at midnight, giving bread to a hungry crowd, or
encouraging a repentant thief.

James N. Lapsley points out how the early church
developed a dualistic divergence between salvation and
health (Lapsley 1972:42, 43) and adds,

From the 16th century to the 20th there was
perhaps a greater dichotomy between salvation
and health among Protestants than at any other
period in Christian history . . . . The body-
soul distinction and the compartmentalization
of the mind, so one aspect of it (feeling or
willing) . . . [has plagued the church until]
in recent years a considerable amount of progress has been made toward understanding the
relationship between salvation and health . . . .
Since about 1950, several astute thinkers (45)
in the church have been devoting their attention to this question.

The church is now rediscovering this wholeness in the
health-salvation relationship.

In order to be absolutely sure that 2,000 years of
dualistic thinking does not confuse my own use of terms
in these pages, it may be helpful to say a word about
how I am employing these terms. I have shown that what
Luke and Jesus and the Bible mean by *health* clearly
includes what Christians mean by *salvation*. I have
stated that what modern readers of the Bible ought to
mean by *salvation* ought to include the physical as well
as the spiritual.

However, it should not be expected of the reader (or
the writer!) that he can do mental gymnastics quite so

easily as to be prepared from now on in this document to
use these words in these technically expanded senses.
Thus I will continue to use *health* when I want to make
sure the reader understands me to include the physical
aspect of health/salvation, and I will use *salvation*
when I want to make sure the reader understands me to
include the spiritual aspect of health/salvation.

Thus, in my opinion, if it were possible, people
ought not to use either of these words as being different from the other. But since they often do, when it
is crucial for me to imply both aspects, I will either
use both words or the hyphenated phrase health-salvation.
In other instances as I speak of "the total health of
every person" or a "holistic health program" I very
definitely imply the full meaning of health-salvation.

HEALTH THROUGH FORGIVENESS

When a paralyzed man was let down through an opened
roof because of the crowd around Jesus, the Lord's
surprising words of healing were, "Your sins are for-
given you, my friend" (Luke 5:20, TEV). For constantly
erring humans these words can be the best news ever.
Illness is so intimately related to the things people
do that sick persons universally wonder what they may
have done wrong -- what mistake or sin they may have
committed -- to make them ill. The feeling of guilt
may not only result from sickness, but by its psychoso-
matic effects also cause it, setting up the vicious
circle of guilt-sickness-more guilt-more sickness.
Jesus not only recognized this kind of self-perpetuating
problem, but attacked it directly. He showed us that
the only cure for human guilt is the forgiveness of God
-- that divine forgiveness is the only way to health and
salvation (wholeness).

God, through the suffering, death, and resurrection
of Christ, cleared the channels of access to himself so
that man's proper relationship with him could be
restored. The fact that a forgiving God cares, says
E. G. Homrighausen, is

. . . the Good News that God has set in motion
in Jesus Christ and in history a liberating action

for man's highest welfare personally and commu-
nally (Homrighausen, 1971).

Here is the Gospel -- the good news of forgiveness and
hope, of salvation and healing.

DELIVERING THE MESSAGE

At the end of his earthly life Jesus told his disciples that in the name of the Messiah "the message
about repentance and the forgiveness of sins must be
preached to all nations" (Luke 24:47, 48, TEV). This
is, in effect, extension education about the health-
salvation relationship -- the message of wholeness.
Luke further records that Jesus told his apostles,
"You will be witnesses for me . . . to the ends of the
earth" (Acts 1:8, TEV).

It is clear that the church exists for those *outside*
its walls -- those who have not yet heard the Good News,
and those who have not believed it. It exists for the
kind of evangelism Jesus was engaged in when, "visiting
all the towns and villages, he taught . . . preached
the Good News . . . and healed people from every kind
of disease and sickness" (Matthew 9:35, TEV).

Gandhi used to say that if missionaries would give
up preaching and only continue their works of education
and healing they could have India at their feet. Gandhi
was deeply concerned for the people of India, but
whether through lack of understanding or by design, he
was asking Christians to deny the very heart of their
commitment and the central purpose of their lives.
That purpose is to use every possible means to deliver
Christ's message for the same reason he gave it --
because *the world needs it*, because it offers the life
of meaning and permanence that every person and
society seeks and which no other religion or philosophy
or political system can provide.

Jesus summed up his work at one time by saying,
" . . . the blind can see, the lame can walk, the
lepers are made clean, the deaf can hear, the dead
are raised to life, and the Good News is preached to

the poor" (Luke 7:22, TEV). The church is thus not only uniquely qualified but obligated by its own reason for being, to translate the love it has received from God into action by sharing the message of health and salvation, by becoming a healing community.

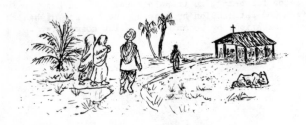

8

THE HEALING COMMUNITY

Doctors and theologians in a World Council of Churches
consultation at Tubingen in 1964 reaffirmed as a
common conviction that

1. the Christian understanding of health is
    unique;

2. the Christian understanding of health and
    healing is intrinsically related to God's
    plan of Salvation; and

3. the Christian ministry of healing belongs
    primarily to the congregation and only in
    this context to those who are profession-
    ally trained in the healing arts.

The church of Jesus Christ has a unique role to fill
as God's agent of constructive change in the midst of
human society. Its task is to heal the world's hurts
and give meaning to all of life. Christians are called
to show and tell how God's saving and healing love
creates new men and women -- what Jesus meant when he

said, "I have come that men may have life, and may have it in all its fullness" (John 10:10b, NEB).

The early Jerusalem church was seriously concerned with the physical needs of its people. "There was not a needy person among them, for as many as were possessors of lands or houses sold them, and brought the proceeds of what was sold and laid it at the apostles' feet; and distribution was made to each as any had need" (Acts 4:34, 35, REV).

The Communists learned their slogan, "From each according to his ability, to each according to his need," from an Anglican person, and thus the Hebrew scriptures and the example of the early church. Virtually every government today has attempted to tax according to people's incomes and use that money to help people in need. But Karl Marx was able to capture the imagination of so many because the church lagged in its concern for the poor and turned a deaf ear to the cries of the exploited during the early days of the Industrial Revolution. Where the church fails to make both health and salvation a part of its task governments take over necessary social services, the church loses its place in the vanguard of social reformation and moral regeneration, and the people lose important dimensions of health care. In Russia, for example, the church is not permitted to speak to social issues, much less to run a health clinic as a sign of its concern for the whole person.

Aware of the church's responsibility for the whole man, missionaries have often involved themselves in activities beyond their commonly understood vocations. Medical missionary David Livingstone strongly condemned the slave traffic. He even translated his concern for Africa's health and salvation into social action by freeing Africans who had been captured to be sold as slaves (Roberts 1875:203). Dr. Marcus Whitman and his associate, Henry Harmon Spalding, added the development of farming and animal husbandry to their efforts for the total health of the Indians of the American Northwest.(46)

In earlier, simpler times missionaries dealt with basic needs, using what tools were available to them.

They preached. They healed. They taught. They
observed, recorded, and wrote. In a simpler age they
were virtually prepared for any problem. They did what
they could and were highly effective in many ways. But
human expectations have grown increasingly complex in
these days of technology and specialization, nationalism
and social consciousness. Now missionaries and other
Christian workers often wonder how their specific skill
fits in and how to be effective in the face of a large
variety of interlocking problems. They also see that
heavily funded government, foundation, and even church
projects have often left developing countries with
imported programs they cannot afford to continue.
Western technology, in solving one specific problem,
may do little good or even create other problems.

In the past few years many of those concerned with
health of the whole person have begun to look critically
at the work of the church and its institutions. They
realize that all our efforts have not stopped the
world from getting sicker. Hospitals and churches
alike have failed to meet the world's needs with a
convincing message of health and salvation. Can
mission institutions provide a service which is adequate and cost-effective? Can the church offer a life
of wholeness in a way that fills and gives meaning to
the good in cultures with differing world views?

TECHNOLOGY AND STEWARDSHIP

"New occasions teach new duties; Time
makes ancient good uncouth...." (47)

It is strange that we Western Christians who so
admire modern technology have often failed to make use
of it in our churches. We have made our plans a year
at a time or in response to current problems and
challenges instead of setting measurable long-range
goals. We have yet to see what could be done if
mission planners were systematically to analyze the
needs of a specific group of people, set a specific
objective of persuading those people to accept the
abundant life Christ offers, and then prepare and carry
out a strategy directed toward this end.

Systems analysis, operations research, data processing, and programming should be used for the Kingdom of God as well as for the business world. We excuse ourselves by saying that the church is not a business, but if the church is to run programs, good stewardship requires us to use every resource available as efficiently and responsibly as we can.

The systems approach to planning requires us to make our observations as complete as possible by means of surveys; formulate the problems and list them in order of priority; verify our assumptions, especially with regard to available resources; determine broad general long-range goals, list specific objectives in priority order; determine measurable short-term goals; develop a strategy; experiment with models by operations research; organize all resources; execute the programs; have results evaluated, preferably by a third party; record and report conclusions; and replan as necessary if goals are not achieved. This is the approach that will keep our attention on what we want to accomplish and help us to avoid getting lost in details that lead us in circles. Let us briefly reflect on our purpose, goals, objectives, and strategy.

Our *purpose* is the purpose of the church: to honor God; to make Jesus Christ known to all as the Savior who heals and gives life and reconciles men to God and each other; to confront each person with the decision to accept Christ as Savior and to become a responsible member of his body, the church; to demonstrate God's love to all through the ministry of teaching and healing which Jesus began. Our aim is, in fact, to offer all people health and salvation.

Our broad, general long-range *goals* are (1) to improve the general level of health through community-oriented health care programs using basic health workers trained and supported by health team resources of mission and other voluntary hospitals or clinics; (2) to implement cost-effective programs of coordinated community health services that will not only affect certain isolated situations, but will also provide models which may profitably be adapted by developing countries for both rural and urban communities; and (3) to have healing communities in each village, hamlet, town, and ghetto.

Each society must become an organism with creative self-giving vital to its life.

Our *objectives* are to train effective basic health workers, establish holistic health centers and develop these centers into healing communities. Where the basic health workers are members of the body of Christ, the healing community may be a church, concerned and involved with the total health of every person.

The health workers, centers, churches, institutions, and back-up agencies must set their own measurable short-term goals. For example, a realistic minimum goal for each Christian institution would be to establish five new health centers annually, at least one and perhaps each of which would become a new church.

Certain guidelines should direct the *strategy* of our holistic health program:

1. It must be faithful to our purpose.

2. It must reach everyone in the target area -- not only those who come to our churches and hospitals.

3. It must be aimed at correcting basic health problems.

4. It must involve the target people in planning and responsibility in order to be relevant to their needs and culture.

5. It must be cost-effective so that it is replicable with local staff and resources.

6. It must be integrated with all other available health programs.

7. It must develop healing communities -- churches or their functional equivalents -- for further health development.

Our most readily available and reliable resource in most areas will be the established mission hospitals. These are the places where physicians have most

effectively exercised their technical skills, faith-
fully healing the sick who have come to them, and have
high esteem among the local people. Mission institutions comprise a large percentage of the total number
of hospital beds in most developing countries. We need
to preserve them and use them to capacity, both in
rural areas where most of the population now lives, and
in urban centers where most people will be living after
a few decades. Public health enthusiasts sometimes
underrate the importance of hospitals, but preventive
and curative medicine are inseparable.

Attached to these institutions we must build modular
systems of coordinated community health services that
reach as far as there are people. This means that
mission health services, instead of contracting, must
expand as rapidly as possible to help meet the need of
developing countries which are as yet unable to cope
with their total health problems.

THE STRATEGY -- HEALING COMMUNITIES

In developing our strategy we need first to clear
the decks of those programs, institutions, and professionals that are not willing or able to participate
in developing healing communities. By continual computer or other objective analysis we must also
challenge every participant to be cost-effective. We
cannot afford to have the kind of system in which, as
one government worker recently said, "They pretend to
pay us, and we pretend to work."

Trained basic health workers who have their own
means of livelihood supplemented on a fee for service
basis from their own communities will not need costly
outside support. However, each health worker should
receive some form of recognition and status appropriate
to his training. The community development committee
must have power to confer status as well as to take
it away in case of poor performance. In effect, these
committees will determine who may be their basic
health workers. The advocate-trainers must respect
the committee's decisions even if those chosen as basic
health workers or leaders are illiterate.(48)

We need to be aware of the potential for conversion and spiritual growth of non-Christian practitioners who are chosen by their communities to be agents of change. At the well in Sychar Jesus talked with a woman whose qualifications for leadership were certainly question-able, yet because of this encounter she became a witness through whom many of her community met Christ (John 4:39-42). On other occasions Jesus used the faith of a Canaanite woman and a Roman centurion for his work of health and salvation (Luke 7:9, 10; Matthew 15:28). Although man, unaided, cannot perfect his own culture and needs help from outside, we can use the knowledge and the good in any culture as a starting point for working toward total health in that society.

At the same time it is clear that total health requires the transforming of certain world views. From the point of view of a Hindu who believes in reincarna-tion, either family planning or the destruction of pests may keep a soul from being reborn. Muslims are family planning as man's attempt to challenge the will of Allah. By inviting and encouraging others to become Christ's disciples, we can point the way to freedom from cyclic and restrictive world views and open the door to achievement of each person's maximum potential. This is evangelism which should lead to the development of indigenous churches -- healing communities which will be the functional equivalent of development committees but with an added dimension.

Smalley defines an indigenous church as

. . . a group of believers who live out their life including their socialized Christian activity, in the pattern of the local society, and for whom any transformation of that society comes out of their felt needs under the guid-ance of the Holy Spirit and the Scriptures (Smalley 1958:55).

The indigenous worshipping and working Christian community then becomes free to be its own kind of center of healing. Each member's special gifts and talents can be fully used for the transformation of society. Pastors, elders, and other church members may be trained by teams from larger institutions in

agriculture, literacy, family planning, public health,
or direct patient care. By developing the local church-
health center teams the institutions extend their
effectiveness over as broad an area as possible.

In a Western context, Granger E. Westberg has success-
fully developed several holistically oriented health
centers in church buildings which have been adapted
appropriately for this purpose.(49) The church-based
health clinic can be run as a non-profit charity organization, supporting itself by a sliding fee for service
that fits the needs of patients. Clerical, pastoral
counseling, and medical staff may be employed, but
volunteers from the church greatly assist in the planning and running of the clinic.

When church buildings are empty most of the week,
using them for this kind of community service is
obviously good stewardship. The church is assisting
the clinic and community while the clinic, by paying
for the use of normally empty facilities, also supports
the church. Other forms of community development and
service can be church-based in the same way, helping
to meet the needs of people around the world.

CAN HOSPITALS BE SELF-SUPPORTING?

Church-based health centers run by healing congrega-
tions in the small community, ghetto, or village need
the back-up and training facilities of a hospital. The
WHO Expert Committee on Organization of Medical Care
describes a hospital as, ideally, an integral part of
a social and medical organization, the function of
which is to provide for the population's complete care,
both curative and preventive, whose out-patient services
reach to the family in its home environment; the
hospital is also a center for the training of health
workers and for bio-social research.

It is possible for a church hospital to be all of
this and still be self-supporting because of its
curative work. Dr. Danial Isaac, General Secretary of
the Christian Medical Association of India, has developed
an excellent paper on the use of cost accounting for
keeping hospital departments solvent and constantly

supportive.(50) Realistic planning and efficient
management are keys to self-support. John D. Rollins
has prepared *An Accounting Guide for Voluntary Hospital*
in India to help managers keep fiscal control of their
institutions.(51) A model hospital financial statement
is included in Appendix C.

Most mission hospitals can be run cheaply because
the public does not demand or expect costly services.
The families of patients often want to feed, bathe,
comfort and care for their loved ones. General hospitals in the U. S. A. keep a staff-patient ratio of
three to one, while mission hospitals can often give
equally good medical care with a staff-patient ratio
of less than one staff member to a patient. Higher
costs of running mission hospitals are usually due to
Western criteria of convenience for staff rather than
the needs or desires of the patients and their families.
Without sacrificing cleanliness or excellence of care,
eye, ear, nose and throat patients, orthopedic,
psychiatric, maternity, tuberculous, and chronically
ill patients can easily be kept in simple, family
assisted units built with inexpensive locally available
and culturally adaptable materials.

Viggo Olsen, a medical missionary in Bangladesh, has
defined a series of principles for medical missions.
One of his observations is that

. . . a hospital in a poor area cannot be
expected to be completely self-supporting, or
charges will be excessive and the poor neglected
in favor of the wealthy (Olsen 1973:350).

In certain circumstances, especially as severe as those
he experienced, it may be impossible for a hospital to
survive without foreign subsidy, but in many situations
assistance from local or central governments and
insurance plans and income from special services may
be available. Those who request and can afford special
services should be required to pay for them and thus
subsidize some of the charity services.

Elite teaching hospitals usually require education
grants. High tuition fees, while they help the institution, penalize capable students from poor families.

Government support and endowments for scholarships or teaching posts are often the only solution.

The most valuable assistance for developing nations that do not yet have enough allied health professionals is the dedicated Christian missionary. Even where their support comes from their home countries, a salary should be paid through the institutions' budgets in national salary scale equivalents so that these budgets represent the total cost of running the institutions, and so the missionary is not irreplaceable for financial reasons alone.

The next most valuable form of assistance is endowments for leadership training and also for services to the poor, but these must be at a level the nation can be expected to match should it wish to duplicate the mission facility in other places. Indeed, this should be one of the goals of all church and mission related medical programs in a country. They should be so organized and administered that they can serve as models for secular agencies to imitate.

Grants for essential equipment and buildings are valuable if they do not add expenses for additional services or maintenance which have no continuing source of support. The annual cost of maintenance or operation of added services is usually over one-fifth of the total initial capital investment. This fact needs to be kept in mind whenever we contemplate installing new facilities, for we are not doing developing nations a favor if we raise their expectations too high by initiating programs that are beyond their financial ability to take over.

THE PLACE OF THE DOCTOR

H. Schwarz of Acha-Tugi Hospital in Cameroun says that church doctors are the wrong people to be in charge of total health Programs. He adds:

> This is not their own fault; they have been
> recruited under quite different circumstances
> . . . . they have been engaged by an appeal
> to their hearts, and thus they are belonging

to a type who by nature is more inclined to
listen to his heart than to follow his intel-
lectual conclusions -- and the heart is
always a short-sighted organ!

The disproportion between human suffering and
available help calls for wise planning to make
the most out of it, to reach an utmost efficiency . . . .

Now, to help us carry out the agreed priority
programs, we have to ask for staff able to
follow these basic arguments . . . . They would
need "more brain and less heart" or at least
the strength of character to have a balanced
control over both . . . .

They are still very much needed in the overall
service, and our instructions with conferences,
pamphlets, study groups have to continue just
to make them aware of the various tasks and
necessary adjustments. But for the real execut-
ing staff one has to select a new type of co-
worker with quite different background, formation
and character (*Contact 13*:15, 16).

Michael Gass of Adiodome, Ghana, agrees with
Schwarz. He writes:

    . . . physicians are not the best category of
people to appoint as directors of community
health or preventive medicine programs -- in
fact, they are almost the last group we should
turn to for filling these posts. I would
hasten to add here that they are, however,
some of the most valuable individuals to use
as advisers and consultants and critics.

Now, let's look at a list of the qualities
and skills and areas of knowledge that are
required of a director of a community health,
public health, preventive medicine or health
care delivery program . . . . This man or
woman should be familiar with the local situation, be politically aware and astute, be
a good economist, be evangelistic, be

culturally sensitive, be sociologically sound,
be experienced in personnel management, be
flexible, be an educationist, be a nutritionist,
be a decision maker, and be familiar with basic
health principles.

. . . . It is my contention that the director
of such a program needs no more medical knowledge than what is taught in the hygiene course
at teacher training college in most developing
countries. If a problem comes up requiring
more technical knowledge than that, he can turn
to his consultant, the friendly district medical
officer.

. . . the group most adapted to the above criteria are experienced teachers in primary and
middle schools. Many developing countries have
been running teacher training colleges for many
years and have graduated a substantial number
of people who are gifted beyond the requirements
of their jobs. They have the great advantage of
being at home in the places we are talking about.
Their qualifications would help them not to fall
into the trap of trying to be all things to all
people (*Contact 13*:17, 18).

This is not to excuse medical doctors from active
participation in comprehensive community health programs, but it should encourage other members of the
allied health professional teams to take more active
management roles. In mission hospitals physicians
often are required to hold the most responsible
positions. We agree with Carl Taylor that the chief
medical officer, medical superintendent, or director
of a hospital should be a part of the community health
team and give active support to the extension program
by periodically visiting basic health workers and
their communities. In general, however, doctors should
be involved at the level of their training and not in
the details of local management.

The doctor's most valuable service may be to help
in the preparation of programmed instruction material
or in liaison with government officials and represen-
tatives of other local development projects. In any

case, medical superintendents or directors should be
totally committed to serving and motivating their
entire staffs to serve in comprehensive community
development programs. A Chinese proverb says: When
you make a person change his thinking, you become
responsible for him. The doctors are in the logical
and also most favorable position to be responsible for
insuring the kind of follow-up community care that
will promote health in all its aspects.

LOOKING FOR LEADERS

Halting and reversing the destructive cycles in
which so many are trapped requires those with special
skills which are the gifts of God and with the love
for Christ that leads to compassion for their fellow-
men. It requires those who are willing to spent time
and effort out of proportion to immediate rewards,
people who have a deep sense of integrity and justice,
people who will work as a team to attack in an integrated way the many problems that must be solved if
the world is ever to achieve health. One of their
tasks will be to recognize and develop the abilities
of others in their communities. Part of our strategy
is to invest in leadership training so that church
leaders will be instructed in theology, psychology,
anthropology, public health -- whatever subjects may
be involved in the total health-salvation relationship

The knowledge and efforts of national church health
workers alone will not be sufficient. There is a law
in the science of development that the effectiveness
of a local program is proportional not to the sum of
the amounts of local and outside effort, but to the
product of personal effort from inside and outside.
The Church is supranational, and all churches in all
nations need missionaries, including those of the
so-called Christian nations and communities who still
have much to learn from the Third World about spiritual maturity.

More missionaries are needed for countries where
national churches have difficulty crossing ethnic,
cultural, language, caste, or prejudice barriers
among their own peoples. Sometimes foreign missionari

can cross these barriers more freely, especially in an
approach to the great ethnic religions -- Islam,
Hinduism, and Buddhism. Yet only 5 to 10 percent of
the present missionary force is devoting full time to
the followers of these religions. A much larger number
will be needed to offer them health and salvation. The
evangelical, supranational, ecumenical, holistically
oriented servant missionary will be needed until

> . . . in honor of the name of Jesus
> All beings in heaven, and on the earth,
>   and in the world below
> Will fall on their knees,
> And all will openly proclaim
>   that Jesus Christ is the Lord
> To the glory of God the Father
>   (Philippians 2:10, 11, TEV).

How can the world hear and be healed unless the
Church sends its messengers of health and salvation?
Because of the diversity of the tasks all kinds of
missionaries are needed. They may be full-time and
fully supported, they may be part-time in a tentmaking
(i.e., self-supporting) ministry, or they may be
volunteers. In spite of a holistic, integrated
approach to planning, some individual missionaries may
have to be professional specialists sent periodically
to accomplish specific tasks.(52)

Many kinds of team relationships can have a part in
the health-salvation strategy. Missionaries may be
under the direction of their sending agencies as well
as depending on them for support, or they may be free
to act independently, or they may be sent by a particular denomination to serve on a different team, as many
American missionaries are sent to serve under national
churches in other countries. The Church Missionary
Society (C. M. S.) is an Anglican team of senders and
sent, administratively independent of any church
structure, although loyal to the Church of England.
Perhaps the ideal team is one in which, as David M.
Stowe suggests, "the members and ministers [of churches
in all countries] should claim each other, and see the
resources of all as resources for a common mission
throughout the world" (Stowe, 1973).

There are a number of organizations concerned for healing through the Body of Christ, the church. One is the *International Order of St. Luke the Physician*, an organization which makes healing a part of the activity of churches wherever they are located.(53)

People of like interests and concerns must encourage and support each other. A new study -- the ethnology of health -- might be created to develop means of relating health and salvation more effectively to the total needs of man. To develop this fully, the highest level of strategy will be an international society for health and salvation along the following lines:

Purpose: To discover and implement ways in which all mankind in every sociocultural group may be reached with the Good News of the possibility of life in all its fullness.

Membership: Allied health professionals, behavioral scientists, anthropologists, theologians, historians, missionaries, and missiologists.

Organization: The structure should be associated or incorporated with organizations having appropriate training and research facilities.(54)

Functions:

1. To accumulate data on the customs, thought patterns, felt needs, health problems, anxieties, religious interests and concerns of each separate culture.

2. To computerize and bank programmed information.

3. To interpret collected data in order to develop effective strategies and workable programs.

4. To consult on ways and means to study and research different sociocultural groups.

5. To publish periodically new research data, strategies, techniques, challenges, opportunities, kinds of training programs, teaching

materials, sources of information, resources, and services.

6. To serve as an information exchange regarding volunteer or career recruitment opportunities and make available all other banked data.

7. To study ways of coordinating health and human development services worldwide and develop guidelines to evaluate their effectiveness.

8. To research financial and other resources for the activities of its members.

9. To develop study seminars and conferences for periodically updating missionary and foreign professionals in promotion of total community health services.

10. To explore theological implications of health and human development programs, their objectives and strategies.

11. To train personnel who will initiate new programs, conduct seminars, and carry on research and consultations as required.

THE CHALLENGE

After developing a strategy our program requires experimenting, organizing, and implementing. We challenge all missionaries, their institutions, their agencies, and Christians throughout the world to be involved.

We have described a modular system of coordinated community health services designed to halt the downward spirals which grip so much of the world. We have suggested a functional and dynamic concept of health which includes salvation -- holistically interrelated means and ends -- relevant to all persons and cultures. Along with examples of a number of programs already in operation, we have offered additional specific suggestions.

Our workable and cost-effective system begins and ends with self-supporting basic health workers in each community who are continually trained and supervised by coordinated development teams from established and firm bases, and assisted by local healing communities.

The church, in all its diversity, still possesses the world's most highly motivated and qualified people. More than all others they should be receptive to the sort of training that will enable them to explain and demonstrate health and salvation, whether as outside advocates of change or as innovators within a community because they are dedicated to sharing, by every means, all that Christ began to do and to teach of life in all its fullness.

APPENDIXES

APPENDIX A

SAMPLE PATIENT CARE RECORD FOR BASIC HEALTH WORKER SUPERVISION
(Symptoms and diagnoses must be changed to those locally appropriate)

NAME OF PATIENT _____ DATE _____

ADDRESS _____ AGE _____

WHY PATIENT CAME _____

Mark with "X" the symptoms or sicknesses that you will treat:

FEVER___ & CHILLS___ & SWEATS___	FLU___ TB___ PNEUMONIA___
COUGH___ & PHLEGM___ & BLOOD___	COLD___ BRONCHITIS___ ASTHMA___
HEADACHE___ STIFF NECK___ CONVULSION___	WHOOPING COUGH___ MEASLES___
DIARRHEA___ & BLOOD___ & MUCOUS___	WORMS (KIND?)___ HEPATITIS___ ANEMIA___
VOMITING___ COLIC___ DISTENSION___	DEHYDRATION___ CONSTIPATION___
SWELLING (WHERE?)___ GLANDS (WHERE?)___	MALNUTRITION___ VITAMIN DEFICIENCY___
URINARY: PAIN___ STONE___ PUS___	URINARY STONE___ VD___ ABSCESS (WHERE?)___
SORE EYES___ TOOTHACHE___ RASH___	SKIN DISEASE (WHERE?)___ INFECTION___
BACKACHE___ JOINT PAIN___	RHEUMATISM: COMMON___ INFLAMED___
HEMORRHAGE: BEFORE___ AFTER___ DELIVERY___	ABORTION: THREATENED___ COMPLETE___
NERVOUSNESS___ DIZZINESS___ FAINT___	IMMUNIZATIONS (WHICH?)___
OTHER SYMPTOMS___	FAMILY PLANNING___ CHILDREN #___

KIND AND DOSE OF MEDICINE	HOW MANY TIMES/DAY	FOR HOW LONG	COST
OTHER TREATMENT GIVEN			

TOTAL _____

ADVICE GIVEN (DIET, HYGIENE, WHEN TO RETURN, etc.) _____

PATIENT BECAME: CURED _____ RELIEVED _____ WORSE _____ OTHER _____

PATIENT WAS SENT TO: HOSPITAL (WHICH?) _____ DOCTOR (WHICH?) _____

WAS PATIENT SENT TO YOU FOR MEDICINE? _____ BY WHOM? _____

REASON IF TREATMENT WAS NOT CARRIED OUT _____

SIGNATURE _____

APPENDIX B

COST-EFFECTIVE MULTIFUNCTIONAL BASIC HEALTH WORKER TRAINING
for Coordinated Holistic Community Health Services by In-Service Extension
Education from Hospitals, Clinics, Colleges, Seminaries, or other Self-
Supporting Institutions under the direction of Area Health Service Teams

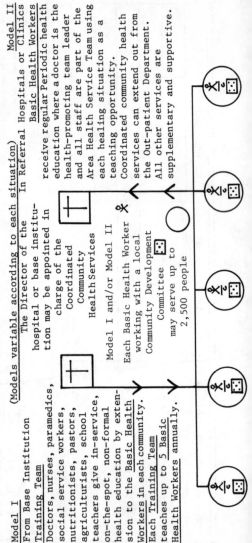

Model I
From Base Institution
Training Team
Doctors, nurses, paramedics,
social service workers,
nutritionists, pastors,
agriculturists, school
teachers give in-service,
on-the-spot, non-formal
health education by extension to the Basic Health
Workers in each community.
Each Training Team
teaches up to 5 Basic
Health Workers annually.

(Models variable according to each situation)

The Director of the
hospital or base institu-
tion may be appointed in
charge of the
Coordinated
Community
Health Services

Model I and/or Model II
Each Basic Health Worker
working with a local
Community Development
Committee
may serve up to
2,500 people

Model II
In Referral Hospitals or Clinics
Basic Health Workers
receive regular periodic health
education where a doctor is the
health-promoting team leader
and all staff are part of the
Area Health Service Team using
each healing situation as a
teaching opportunity.
Coordinated community health
services can extend out from
the Out-patient Department.
All other services are
supplementary and supportive.

Coordinated Community Development and Health Services will need to have the cooperation of Village or Ghetto Councils, Social or Religious Power Structure, Tribal Chiefs, etc.

Basic Health Workers locally chosen, sanctioned, possibly supported (or self-supported) will be multifunctional agents of change for health who learn to instruct and motivate others, are supervised by Community Development Committees, visited at least weekly by the Director, constantly updated, possibly even trained to basic registerable levels, and may become equipped for:

Health surveys; case finding; follow-up (leprosy, tbc., etc.); referrals; liaison; school health programs; adult literacy; evangelism; family welfare planning; first aid; home deliveries; day care centers; immunizations; well baby clinics; prenatal and postnatal care; community health education; low cost self-supporting agricultural demonstrations; "employment-generating low-capital development projects; instruction in nutrition; labor-intensive small scale industrial programs; self-help, self-financing social service facilities; poultry farms; fish culture; animal husbandry; sanitation instruction; dental prophylaxis and care; maintenance of family files; symptomatic treatment; possibly even routinized curative treatment (under appropriate medical supervision) for minor illnesses, i.e., simple diarrhea, bronchitis, malaria, etc., with complete and accurate records to assure quality control by periodic evaluation.

Holistic development programs help people to, in a self-sustaining way, control or cope with their environments (internal and external) so that by physical, mental, social, and spiritual integration they may achieve the maximum potential in all of human life.

APPENDIX C

HOSPITAL FINANCIAL STATEMENT

Period of Report for the year: From _____ 19___ To _____ 19___

Name of Institution _____

Location _____

Income		Expense	
Gross Patient Fees	____	Administration	____
Less Free Care	____	Property & Motor (Autos)	____
Net Patient Fees	____	Housekeeping & Linen	____
% Charity Given	____	Laundry	____
Grants – Pres. Commission	____	Stores	____
– Other	____	Food	____
Gifts – Foreign	____	Prof. Care Patients:	
– Local	____	Doctors Salaries	____
Other Income	____	Nurses Salaries	____
		Other Salaries	____
		Drugs	____
		Med.-Surg. Supplies	____
		Other Expenses	____
		Nurses Training School	____
		Hosp. Children	____
		Rural Dispensary	____
		Prov. for Depreciation	____
		Other Expense	____
		TOTAL EXPENSE	____
		GAIN (LOSS)	____
TOTAL INCOME	____		

Financial Indicators

Net Patient Fees/Pt-Day	_____
All Other Income/Pt-Day	_____
Total Income/Pt-Day	_____
Total Expenses/Pt-Day	_____
GAIN (LOSS)/Pt-Day	_____

Indoor		
	– Admissions	_____
	– Total Patients Day Care	_____
	– Avg. Daily Census	_____
	– Bed Capacity	_____
	– % Bed Occupancy	_____
Outdoor	– New Patients	_____
	– Old Patients	_____
	– Total Visits	_____
	– % Charity Given	_____

BALANCE SHEET

Assets	
Cash	_____
Investments	_____
Inventories	_____
Other Assets	_____
TOTAL ASSETS	_____

Liabilities	
Accounts Payable	_____
Employee Deposits	_____
Special Funds	_____
Plant Funds	_____
Reserves for Depreciation	_____
Other Liabilities	_____

Net Worth	
Opening Balance	_____
Gain (Loss)	_____
TOTAL LIABILITIES & NET WORTH	_____

SIGNED _____

Dispensaries or clinics:

a. _____
b. _____
c. _____
d. _____
e. _____
f. _____

NOTES

1. We are indebted for many of the facts which we are incorporating into the concept of interrelated self-perpetuating cycles to Lester R. Brown in his book *World Without Borders* and to Random House which gave permission for the use of his material.

2. This list is compiled from p. 389 of *New Perspectives in Cultural Anthropology* by Roger M. and Felix M. Keesing and from p. 173 of *The Church and Cultures* by Louis J. Luzbetak.

3. Anthony F. C. Wallace calls this world view "basic beliefs and values"; Nida, the "system of values"; and A. R. Tippett equates it with "religion."

4. Compiled from pp. 257ff. of Luzbetak's *Church and Cultures* and from Foster's *Traditional Societies and Technological Change*, pp. 151ff.

5. See Gunawan Nugroho's *Community Health Insurance Scheme*, Panti Walujo Hospital, Solo, Central Java, 1972. Also helpful are pp. 603-627 of "The Kojedo

Project and Community Medicine," a Description of
the Kojedo Community Health and Development Project
Shil Jun Lee, Ha Chung Myun, Kojedo, Kyung Nam,
Korea. The Director of this project is John R.
Sibley, and the Associate Director is J. J. Kim
(p. 17).

6. Winter in *Theological Education by Extension*, pp.
    308 and 309, speaks of the advantages of theological
    education by extension in the worker's own local
    environment. The same applies to health education.

7. For excellent Baseline Survey Forms see *Planning
    Community Health Programmes* by Esther G. Mabry,
    M.C., M.P.H., published by the Christian Medical
    Association of India in 1972.

8. Two excellent books on this subject are *A Guide to
    Health Education in Leprosy* by P. J. Neville,
    M.A.O.T., and D. Ottaway (available from the All
    Africa Leprosy and Rehabilitation Training Centre,
    Addis Ababa, Ethiopia) and the *Reference and Train-
    ing Manual for the Physical Therapy Technicians in
    Leprosy* by Judith Pasnik, R.P.T., and Oliver W.
    Hasselblad, M.D. (available from American Leprosy
    Missions, Inc., in New York).

9. See April Allison Kawacki's *A Textbook for Family
    Planning Field Workers*, Community and Family Study
    Center, University of Chicago, 1971.

10. For simple but complete training in first aid by
    programmed instruction see the American National
    Red Cross's four-volume *Basic First Aid* (Garden
    City, N.Y.: Doubleday and Company, Inc., 1971) and
    the Boy Scouts of America's *First Aid* (New Brunswic
    N.J., 1973).

11. See chapter 17, "Immunizing the Under-Fives" by
    Paget Stanfield in *Medical Care in Developing
    Countries*, edited by Maurice King.

12. See chapter 16, "The Under-Fives Clinic" by David
    Morley, in *Medical Care in Developing Countries*,
    edited by Maurice King.

13. See *You and Your Baby* by Mrs. M. Kiyvenhoven, S.R.N., S.C.M., and B. D. Siddique, (Gujranwala, Pakistan: Nirali Kitaben, 1972).

14. An excellent book is *Nutrition for Developing Countries* by Maurice and Felicity King, David Morley, and Leslie and Ann Burgess (London: Oxford University Press, 1972). It is also available from Oxford Press in Nairobi, Dar es Salaam, Lusaka, and Addis Ababa.

15. A good study of water resources development is found on pages 1-143 of Village Technology Handbook produced by VITA (Volunteers for International Technical Assistance) and published by the College Campus, Schenectady, N.Y. in 1970.

16. See David Morley's "Medical Records," chapter 26 in *Medical Care in Developing Countries*, edited by Maurice King.

17. See pages 145-181 of *Village Technology Handbook* by VITA.

18. See Maurice King's "The Laboratory," chapter 24 in *Medical Care in Developing Countries*, edited by Maurice King.

19. I would recommend Daniel E. Fountain's *The Art of Diagnosis for Medical Assistants*, C.B.Z.O. - Vanga, B. P. 4728, Kinshasa 2, Zaire.

20. Three books I have found to be very helpful in this area:

    Symptom-Treatment Manual by B. Bajracharya, M.B.B.S. and M. Bomgaars, M.D., M.P.H. (Shanta Bhawan Community Health Program, Kathmandu, Nepal, 1973).

    "Material Aids for Teaching Rural Para-Medical Workers" by Joseph A. Narke and available from the Behrhorst Clinic and Hospital of Chimaltenango, Guatemala.

    The Field Worker's Medical Manual, produced by the Summer Institute of Linguistics, Inc. in 1973 and

available from the Wycliffe Bible Translators, Inc.,
Box 1960, Santa Ana, Calif. 92702.

21. Dr. Carroll Behrhorst has developed a simple and
    useful record for each patient visit. In addition
    to a definite and limited list of diseases which
    promotores are permitted to treat initially, there
    are spaces for noting all details about medications
    or advice given and charges made.

22. It is reported that manic depression is frequent
    in Denmark but rare in Newfoundland or among
    African Negroes; obsessive neuroses are rare in
    Taiwan, Kenya, and Kuwait; conversion hysteria is
    common in Ireland, Greece, and Italy; psychosomatic
    disorders are fewer and less intractable in Ireland
    than in most other places, but are especially prom-
    inent among migrant populations; homosexuality is
    rare in Hong Kong but more frequent in Iran and
    Brazil; schizophrenia, which apparently is ubiqui-
    tous, is quieter in developing countries than in
    the Western world (E. D. Wiltkower and J. Friend
    in *Culture and Mental Health*, edited by Marvin
    Kaufmann Opler, MacMillan, 1959, pp. 492, 496).

23. Communities in the Western world tend to reject
    these patients and "put them away" in institutions
    out of fear, ignorance, and guilt. This deperson-
    alizes the patients and makes recovery much more
    difficult. Often when patients in institutions
    have an operation or die, the relatives, although
    they have been notified, do not care or dare to
    come to the hospital (personal comments by the
    Rev. Carl J. Rote, Chaplain of Letchworth Village,
    Stony Point, N.Y., and the Rev. C. H. Hazlett).
    This is because of an insecurity about their own
    mental integrity when the "borderline between
    'abnormal' and 'normal' is vague and arbitrary"
    (John and Elaine Cumming in Paul and Miller 1955:
    48).

24. This possibility is present in all kinds of socie-
    ties and the death wish, whether internalized or
    projected, may be evident or completely buried in
    the subconscious.

25. World Neighbors has produced a filmstrip entitled "How to Take Soil Samples for Analysis." It is available from World Neighbors, 5116 North Portland, Oklahoma City, Okla. 73112.

26. The VITA *Village Technology Handbook* has a very good section on irrigation, pages 185-226.

27. World Neighbors has also produced a filmstrip entitled "Fish Farming for Food and Profit" which I would recommend. See address in Note #25 above.

28. The VITA *Village Technology Handbook* has a good section on this subject on pages 250 to 281.

29. World Neighbors periodically publishes "Soundings" which serves as an idea exchange pamphlet for development of rural industries and other projects. They have catalogs on teaching materials for many kinds of rural development programs, especially through the use of filmstrips.

30. It has been proposed that a curriculum of study for non-literates could be prepared on cassette tapes. Such a curriculum might include: Introduction to Old Testament, Introduction to New Testament, Literacy, Christian Life, Sanitation, Nutrition, Infant Care and Feeding, Community Development, etc. Some Bible studies on tapes are already available. Cassettes and locally prepared printed materials should be kept in waterproof and verminproof containers which can be easily carried.

31. This verse has a special meaning to former outcastes in India who have become Christians. It was Gandhi who called all outcastes "harijans" (God's people).

32. Religious instruction or "Theological Education by Extension" can include teaching the Bible; God's activity in human history; the meaning of Jesus Christ; basic Christian beliefs; pastoral psychology and counseling; appropriate indigenous forms of worship vis-a-vis syncretism; how to establish self-governing, self-propagating, self-supporting churches; and Christian acts of compassionate service.

33. See *Contact 13* (February 1973) and *Contact 15* (June 1973) put out by the Christian Medical Commission of the World Council of Churches, 150 Route de Ferney, 1211 Geneva 20, Switzerland.

34. For the story of Carroll Behrhorst, see *Physician to the Mayas* by Edward Barton (Philadelphia: Fortress Press, 1970).

35. Joseph A. Narke, a Peace-Corps volunteer, wrote this manual entitled "Material Aids for Teaching Rural Para-Medical Workers." It is available from the Behrhorst Clinic and Hospital, Chilmaltenango, Guatemala, C.A.

36. World Neighbors, founded by John Peters, has effectively supported and directed the agricultural program associated with the Behrhorst Clinic and Hospital.

37. Dr. Eugene H. Evans started the Miraj Village Service over fifteen years ago. This is the program from which Eric Ram, D.P.H., has developed the much larger project.

38. The designation "Integrated Auxiliary Nurse-Midwife" is given to differentiate A.N.M.'s who have completed the integrated training in this program from the regular government-recognized A.N.M.'s not yet trained for this program.

39. See also "We Rejoice in the Hope We Share" by Jane Day Mook, *A. D. Magazine*, October, 1971.

40. Fifteen years ago Dr. and Mrs. Leonard Blickenstaff, at their Rural Public Health Center, developed a multipurpose village worker program which principally combined medical and agricultural functions for improvement of rural life around Anklesvar, Broach District, Gujarat State, India.

41. It is important that the basic health worker be backed up by the predominant power structure with which each community identified. The power may not be invested in the chief person, even if he

is elected to that position. It may be in a
religious, political, social, economic, tribal,
or other cultural structure.

42. The Technical Assistance Information Clearing
House (TAICH) of the American Council of Voluntary
Agencies for Foreign Service, Inc., (200 Park
Avenue South, New York, N.Y. 10003) publishes
directories which contain essential information
describing the activities of U. S. voluntary
agencies, missions, and foundations involved in
overseas development assistance. TAICH can help
the Field Director a great deal.

43. The Rev. Gary W. Demarest, La Canada Presbyterian
Church, La Canada, California.

44. Arthur F. Glasser discusses this subject on page 3
of his unpublished manuscript "Communism and
Evangelical Christianity" which is available from
the author by writing to him at 135 North Oakland,
Pasadena, California 91101. See also Friedrich
Engels' "Ludwig Feuerbach," in *A Handbook of
Marxism* edited by Emile Burns, pages 222-224 (New
York: International Publishers, 1935).

45. Seward Hiltner is among those to whom we are most
indebted.

46. For further discussion of this subject, see p. 185
of Clifford Merril Drury's *Henry Harmon Spalding*
(Caldwell, Idaho: The Caxton Printers, Ltd., 1936)
and p. 230 of William A. Mowry's *Marcus Whitman*
(New York: Silver, Burdett and Co., 1901).

47. From the hymn "Once to Every Man and Nation"
written in 1845 by James Russell Lowell.

48. Two-thirds of the church members in India are
illiterate, but health workers may have to be
chosen from among these. When faced with the
problem of bringing adults up to higher educational
levels, the church in Guatemala had a single book
written in each of the five required subjects.
These books succeeded in helping adults meet

government requirements for training programs. A
number of basic programmed instruction materials
may be obtained from AEBICAM, P. O. Box 131, Choma,
Zambia.

49.   Information on the organization of church-based
health clinics is available from Granger E. Westber
Wholistic Health Center, Inc., 137 S. Garfield Ave.
Hinsdale, Illinois 60521.

50.   Daniel Isaac, Council Lodge, Nagpur 440 001,
Maharashtra, India.

51.   A copy may be obtained from John D. Rollins,
Christian Medical College Hospital, Ludhiana,
Punjab, India.

52.   An excellent service for discovering whether a
person's talents and spiritual gifts are needed
locally or abroad is Intercristo, Box 9323, Seattle
Washington 98109.

53.   Headquarters of the International Order of St.
Luke the Physician is at 2243 Front Street, San
Diego, Calif. 92101.

54.   Such organizations might be The American Society
of Missiology (Gerald Anderson, Ventnor, New
Jersey); The School of World Mission at Fuller
Theological Seminary (135 North Oakland, Pasadena,
Calif. 91101); William Carey Institute, (1021 E.
Walnut, Suite 204, Pasadena, California).

BIBLIOGRAPHY

ALMQUIST, L. Arden. "Medicine and Religion--A Missionary Perspective," *Occasional Bulletin*, New York: Missionary Research Library, April 1967.

ANDERSON, Michael D. "Mission Is Possible: A Bible Study on Mission for Discovery and Response," Presbyterian Distribution Service, 225 Varick Street, New York, N.Y. 10014.

BENEDICT, Ruth. *Patterns of Culture*, New York: Mentor Books, 1934.

BLAIKLOCK, E. M. *St. Luke*, (Scripture Union Bible Study Books), Grand Rapids, Michigan: Wm. B. Eerdmans, 1968.

BROWN, Lester R. *World Without Borders*, New York: Random House, 1972.

BRYANT, John H.
      1969. *Health and the Developing World*, Ithaca: Cornell University Press.

1970. "Moral Issues in Health Care Delivery," Christian Medical Commission, W. C. C., Report of Annual Meeting.

CHRISTIAN LITERATURE SOCIETY FOR CHINA
1917. *China Mission Year Book*, Shanghai.
1924. *China Mission Year Book*.

CHRISTIAN MEDICAL COMMISSION
Contact 13, February 1973, World Council of Churches 150 Route de Ferney, 1211 Geneva 20, Switzerland.
Contact 15, June 1973. World Council of Churches, 150 Route de Ferney, 1211 Geneva 20, Switzerland.

DIEHL, Carl Gustov. "Welfare Work in the Church's Mission," Commission of World Mission, 17th Annual Meeting, Jerusalem, Jordan, April 1965.

DODD, Edward M. "Medical Education," *Educational Year Book*, International Institute of Teacher's College, Columbia University, 1933.

DONNE, John. *Devotions XVII*, quoted in Bold, Robert Cecil, *John Donne, a Life*, New York: Oxford University Press, 1970.

ELLIOTT, Katherine. "Using Medical Auxiliaries: Some Ideas and Examples," *Contact 11*, Geneva: Christian Medical Commission, World Council of Churches, October, 1972.

ENGELS, Friedrich. "Ludwig Feuerbach," *A Handbook of Marxism* (Burns, Emile, ed.), New York: International Publishers, 1935.

FLETCHER, Joseph. *Morals and Medicine*, Boston: Beacon Press, 1954.

FOSTER, George M. *Traditional Societies and Technological Change* (2nd ed.), New York: Harper and Row, 1973.

FREUDENBERGER, C. Dean. "Rural Development and the Christian Churches" (a paper), New York, 1972.

GOLDSCHMIDT, Walter. "Comparative Functionalism: an Essay in Anthropological Theory," Berkeley: University of California Press, 1966, quoted by Kraft, Charles H., in *Dynamic Theologizing*, pre-publication draft, Pasadena, California, 1973.

HESS, Mahlon M. "Political Systems and African Church Polity," *Practical Anthropology*, Vol. 4, No. 5, 1947.

HOMRIGHAUSEN, E. G. "Guidelines Are Needed," *Outlook*, January 11, 1971.

HORN, Joshua S. *Away With All Pests*, New York: Monthly Review Press, 1969.

KESSING, Roger M. and KESSING, Felix M. *New Perspectives in Cultural Anthropology*, New York: Holt, Rinehart and Winston, Inc., 1971.

KING, Maurice, editor. *Medical Care in Developing Countries*, London: Oxford University Press, 1968.

KJAERLAND, Gunnar. "Communicating the Gospel to Illiterate Nomads" in *God, Man and Church Growth*, edited by A. R. Tippett, Grand Rapids, Michigan: William B. Eerdmans, 1973.

KRAFT, Charles. *Dynamic Theologizing*, pre-publication draft, Fuller Theological Seminary, Pasadena, Calif., 1973.

LAPSLEY, James N. *Salvation and Health: The Interlocking Processes of Life*, Philadelphia: Westminster Press, 1972.

LATOURETTE, Kenneth Scott. *A History of Christianity*, New York: Harper and Brothers, 1943.

LENOX HILL HOSPITAL. *Community Outreach News Digest*, New York, August, 1973.

LUZBETAK, Louis J. *The Church and Cultures*, Techny, Illinois: Divine Word Publications, 1970, reprint available from the William Carey Library, South Pasadena, Calif., 1975.

McNAMARA, Robert S. "The Moral Case for Helping the
    World's Poor," Los Angeles Times, 28 September 1973.
    From a report given by McNamara, President of the
    World Bank, to its Board of Governors meeting in
    Nairobi, Kenya, 24 September 1973.

MARTIN, John. "WHO's Endeavour for Better Health,"
    written on the occasion of the 25th anniversary of
    the World Health Organization for World Health Day,
    7 April 1973.

NARKE, Joseph A. "Material Aids to Teaching Rural
    Para-Medical Workers," available from the Behrhorst
    Clinic and Hospital of Chimaltenango, Guatemala.

NIDA, Eugene A. Message and Mission, New York: Harper
    and Row, 1960. Now available from the William Carey
    Library, South Pasadena, Calif.

NUGROHO, Gunawan. Community Health Insurance Scheme,
    Panti Walujo Hospital, Solo, Central Java, 1972.

PADDOCK, William and PADDOCK, Elizabeth. We Don't Know
    How, Ames, Iowa: Iowa State University Press, 1973.

PAUL, Benjamin D. and MILLER, Walter B. Health Culture
    and Community, New York: Russell Sage Foundation,
    1955.

SAI, Fred T. "Defining Health Needs, Health Care
    Priorities and Standards of Health Care." Paper
    prepared for the International Health Conference
    sponsored by the National Council for International
    Health, Washington, D.C., April 25-28, 1973.

STOWE, David M. "1972 in Context," United Church Board
    for World Ministries, 162nd Annual Report, New York,
    January 1, 1973.

SMART, James D. "The Language Problem in Evangelism,"
    Occasional Papers Division of Evangelism, Board of
    National Missions, United Presbyterian Church in
    the U. S. A.

THURBER, David, editor. "The Kojedo Project and Communi
    Medicine," a description of the Kojedo Community

Health and Development Project, Shil Jun Lee, Ha
Chung Myun, Kojedo, Kyung Nam, Korea (John B. Sibley,
Director, J. J. Kim, Associate Director).

UNITED PRESBYTERIAN CHURCH IN THE U. S. A., Board of
National Missions, Division of Evangelism. "A
Study of Some Growing Churches in the U. P. C.,
U. S. A.", May, 1971.

VITA (Volunteers for International Technical Assistance).
Village Technology Handbook. Schenectady, New York:
College Campus, 1970.

WHO EXECUTIVE BOARD REPORT. "Methods of Promoting the
Development of Basic Health Services," submitted to
the 26th World Health Assembly. Reprint from *WHO
Chronicle* No. 7-8, Vol. 27, July-August 1973, for
the Christian Medical Commission, W. C. C.

WINTER, Ralph D., editor. *Theological Education by
Extension*, South Pasadena, Calif.: William Carey
Library, 1969.

ABOUT THE AUTHORS

RONALD SEATON was born in China, the son of missionary parents. He is a graduate of the Johns Hopkins University School of Medicine and a Diplomate of the American Board of Surgery. His surgical residency was interrupted by a period as head of the surgical service in the U. S. Army Field Hospital for prisoners of war in Kojedo, Korea. As a medical missionary in India, he has served as surgeon and as Medical Superintendent of St. Luke's Hospital in Vengurla, and as Director of four Kolhapur Church Council hospitals. In 1970 the United Presbyterian Church called him back to New York to serve as Director of the Office of Health Affairs with responsibility for the United Presbyterian medical work in the United States and abroad. He is a Fellow of the American College of Surgeons, has been a member of the Christian Medical Commission of the World Council of Churches and the National Council for International Health, and was for some time Clinical Assistant Professor of Surgery at the New York Medical College in New York City.

EDITH SEATON is a graduate of the College of Wooster, Wooster, Ohio. In Vengurla, India, she serves as hospital secretary and manager of a home for healthy

children of parents with leprosy. For a time she
edited *Western India Notes*, a magazine published by
the Kolhapur Church Council of the United Church of
North India.

In 1974 the Seatons returned to India where they are
serving the Church of North India under joint appoint-
ment by the United Presbyterian Church, the United
Church of Christ, and the Christian Church (Disciples
of Christ). In addition to his work in St. Luke's
Hospital, Vengurla, Dr. Seaton has instituted community
health programs and training of basic health workers in
nearby villages.

BOOKS BY THE WILLIAM CAREY LIBRARY

GENERAL

The Birth of Missions in America by Charles L. Chaney, $7.95 paper, 352 pp.

Education of Missionaries' Children: The Neglected Dimension of World Mission by D. Bruce Lockerbie, $1.95 paper, 76 pp.

God's Word in Man's Language by Eugene A. Nida, $2.95 paper, 192 pp.

The Holdeman People: The Church in Christ, Mennonite, 1859-1969 by Clarence Hiebert, $17.95 cloth, 688 pp.

Manual for Missionaries on Furlough by Marjorie Collins, $2.95 paper, 160 pp.

The 25 Unbelievable Years: 1945-1969 by Ralph D. Winter, $2.95 paper, 128 pp.

STRATEGY OF MISSION

Church Growth and Christian Mission by Donald A. McGavran, $4.95x paper, pp.

Church Growth and Group Conversion by Donald A. McGavran et al., $2.45 256 pp.

Everything You Need to Grow a Messianic Synagogue by Phillip E. Goble, $2.45 paper, 176 pp.

Growth and Life in the Local Church by H. Boone Porter, $2.95 paper, 124 pp.

A Manual for Church Growth Surveys by Ebbie C. Smith, $3.95 paper, 144 pp.

Reaching the Unreached by Edward C. Pentecost, $5.95 paper, 256 pp.

AREA AND CASE STUDIES

Aspects of Pacific Ethnohistory by Alan R. Tippett, $3.95 paper, 216 pp.

The Baha'i Faith: Its History and Teachings by William M. Miller, $8.95 paper, 450 pp.

A Century of Growth: The Kachin Baptist Church of Burma by Herman Tegenfeldt, $9.95 cloth, 540 pp.

Christ Confronts India by B.V. Subbamma, $4.95 paper, 238 pp.

Church Growth in Japan by Tetsunao Yamamori, $4.95 paper, 184 pp.

Church Planting in Uganda: A Comparative Study by Gailyn Van Rheenen, $4.95 paper, 192 pp.

Circle of Harmony: A Case Study in Popular Japanese Buddhism by Kenneth J. Dale, $4.95 paper, 238 pp.

The Founding and Developing of Spanish Bible Institutes and Seminaries by Janie Marie True, $8.95x paper, 208 pp.

People Movements in the Punjab by Margaret and Frederick Stock, $8.95 paper, 388 pp.

Protestants in Modern Spain: The Struggle for Religious Pluralism by Dale G. Vought, $3.45 paper, 168 pp.

The Religious Dimension in Hispanic Los Angeles by Clifton L. Holland, $9.95 paper, 550 pp.

The Role of the Faith Mission: A Brazilian Case Study by Fred Edwards, $3.45 paper, 176 pp.

Solomon Islands Christianity: A Study in Growth and Obstruction by Alan R. Tippett, $5.95x paper, 432 pp.

Taiwan: Mainline Versus Independent Church Growth by Allen J. Swanson, $3.95 paper, 300 pp.

Tonga Christianity by Stanford Shewmaker, $3.45 paper, 164 pp.

Understanding Latin Americans by Eugene A. Nida, $3.95 paper, 176 pp.

A Yankee Reformer in Chile: The Life and Works of David Trumbull by Irven Paul, $3.95 paper, 172 pp.

THEOLOGICAL EDUCATION BY EXTENSION

Principios del Crecimiento de la Iglesia by Wayne C. Weld and Donald A. McGavran, $3.95 paper, 448 pp.

Principles of Church Growth by Wayne C. Weld and Donald A. McGavran, $4.95x paper, 400 pp.

Theological Education by Extension (revised edition) edited by Ralph D. Winter, $9.95 paper, 656 pp.

The World Directory of Theological Education by Extension by Wayne C. Weld, $5.95x paper, 416 pp. *1976 Supplement only*, $1.95x, 64 pp.

Writing for Theological Education by Extension by Lois McKinney, $1.45x, 64 pp.

APPLIED ANTHROPOLOGY

Becoming Bilingual: A Guide to Language Learning by Donald Larson and William A. Smalley, $5.95x paper, 426 pp.

Christopaganism or Indigenous Christianity? edited by Tetsunao Yamamori and Charles R. Taber, $5.95 paper, 242 pp.

The Church and Cultures: Applied Anthropology for the Religious Worker by Louis J. Luzbetak, $5.95x paper, 448 pp.

Culture and Human Values: Christian Intervention in Anthropological Perspective (writings of Jacob Loewen) edited by William A. Smalley, $5.95 paper, 466 pp.

Customs and Cultures: Anthropology for Christian Missions by Eugene A. Nida, $3.95x paper, 322 pp.

Manual of Articulatory Phonetics by William A. Smalley, $4.95x paper, 522 pp.

Message and Mission: The Communication of the Christian Faith by Eugene A. Nida, $3.95x, 254 pp.

Readings in Missionary Anthropology edited by William A. Smalley, $4.95x paper, 384 pp.

REFERENCE

An American Directory of Schools and Colleges Offering Missionary Courses edited by Glenn Schwartz, $5.95x paper, 266 pp.

Bibliography for Cross-Cultural Workers edited by Alan R. Tippett, $4.95 paper, 256 pp.

Church Growth Bulletin Vols. I-V edited by Donald A. McGavran, $4.95 paper, $6.96 cloth, 404 pp.

Evangelical Missions Quarterly Vols. 7-9, $8.95 cloth, 330 pp.

The Means of World Evangelization: Missiological Education at the Fuller School of World Mission edited by Alvin Martin, $9.95 paper, 544 pp.

The World Directory of Mission-Related Educational Institutions edited by Ted Ward and Raymond Buker, Sr., $19.95x cloth, 906 pp.